Hypertension

A Clinician's Guide
to Diagnosis
and Treatment

Second Edition

Hypertension

A Clinician's Guide to Diagnosis and Treatment

Second Edition

BARRY J. SOBEL, M.D., FACP
Medical Director
Encino Hypertension Center
Encino, California

GEORGE L. BAKRIS, M.D., FACP
Associate Professor of Preventive
  and Internal Medicine
Director, Hypertension/Clinical Research Center
Rush Medical College of Rush University
Rush Presbyterian/St. Luke's Medical Center
Chicago, Illinois

HANLEY & BELFUS, INC./ Philadelphia

Publisher: HANLEY & BELFUS, INC.
                 Medical Publishers
                 210 South 13th Street
                 Philadelphia, PA 19107
                 (215) 546-7293
                 FAX (215) 790-9330
                 Web site: http://www.hanleyandbelfus.com

Library of Congress Cataloging-in-Publication Data

Hypertension : a clinician's guide to diagnosis and treatment / edited
  by Barry Sobel, George L. Bakris. — 2nd ed.
     p.   cm.
  Includes bibliographical references and index.
  ISBN 1-56053-319-6 (alk. paper)
  1. Hypertension Outlines, syllabi, etc. I. Sobel, Barry J.,
1951–   . II. Bakris, George L., 1952–   .
  [DNLM: 1. Hypertension—diagnosis Outlines.
2. Hypertension—therapy Outlines.   WG 18.2 H998 1999]
RC685.H8H7678   1999
616.1'32—dc21
DNLM/DLC
for Library of Congress   99-14490
                                               CIP

**HYPERTENSION: A CLINICIAN'S GUIDE
TO DIAGNOSIS AND TREATMENT, 2nd edition**   ISBN 1-56053-319-6

© 1999 by Hanley & Belfus, Inc. All rights reserved. No part of this book may be repro-
duced, reused, republished, or transmitted in any form or by any means, or stored in a
data base or electronic retrieval system, without written permission of the publisher.

Library of Congress catalog card number 99-14490

Last digit is the print number: 9   8   7   6   5   4

Dedication

To our families

Contents

Preface

This book was written for the busy clinician. It was designed to serve as a quick and up-to-date reference for physicians who evaluate and treat patients with essential and secondary hypertension. In fact, new information is included up until the very week the book goes to press. The new manuscript was initially developed by one of the authors (BJS) to answer questions posed by clinicians at various symposia and lectures. With the aid of the coauthor, it subsequently grew into a book designed to meet the needs of clinicians who do not have time to look up specific clinical questions related to hypertension in encyclopedic textbooks.

This new edition incorporates all the recent advances in the treatment of hypertension in an accessible, quick and easy reference Numerous tables and appendices provide valuable current information on diagnosis, treatment options, medications, dosages, side effects, and more. The text also provides recent references for detailed information about specific topics. We trust you will find this approach useful and welcome suggestions from readers for the next edition.

Barry J. Sobel, M.D., FACP
George L. Bakris, M.D., FACP

Acknowledgments

The authors would like to thank those clinicians and faculty members who have reviewed the manuscript. We would also like to gratefully acknowledge the considerable assistance of Ms. Alexis J. Sobel in the preparation of this second edition.

CHAPTER 1

Clinical Physiology and Pharmacology of Blood Pressure Control

I. **Clinical Physiology of Hypertension: A Clinician's Outline**

   A. **Factors responsible for arterial blood pressure** (Fig. 1)

      1. Blood pressure is determined by **cardiac output** and **peripheral resistance**

      2. Cardiac output depends on **heart rate** and **stroke volume**

         a. **Heart rate** is governed by

            i. **Beta-1 receptors** stimulated by the sympathetic nerves

            ii. **Cholinergic receptors** governed by the parasympathetic nerves

         b. **Stroke volume** is determined by

            i. **Force of contraction** (also influenced by autonomic stimuli)

            ii. **Filling pressure** determined by

               (a) **Venous capacitance**

               (b) **Intravascular fluid volume**

      3. Both peripheral resistance and intravascular fluid volume are influenced by **neural, humoral,** and **renal** factors

         a. Renal mechanisms are responsible for long-term maintenance of arterial pressure, whereas neural mechanisms are responsible for immediate (though less complete) regulation

         b. When the arterial setpoint is abnormally high, the renal-fluid mechanism maintains that level and prevents unlimited long-term increases in arterial pressure

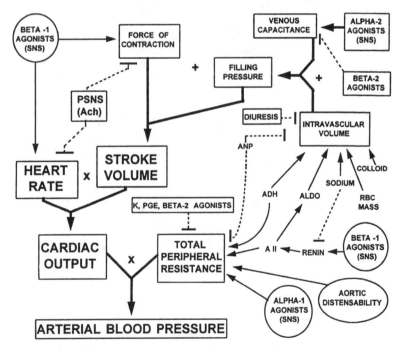

FIGURE 1. Factors responsible for arterial blood pressure. SNS = sympathetic nervous system; PNS = parasympathetic nervous system; Ach = acetylcholine; RBC = red blood cell; ADH = antidiuretic hormone; ALDO = aldosterone; → = stimulatory (positive) influence; - - - ‖ = inhibitory (negative) influence; AI = angiotensin I; AII = angiotensin II; ANP = atrial natriuretic peptide; K = potassium; PGE = prostaglandin E.

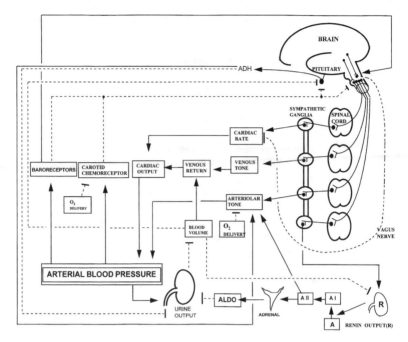

FIGURE 2. Feedback mechanisms in the control of blood pressure. A = angiotensinogen; AI = angiotensin I; AII = angiotensin II; O_2 = oxygen; ADH = antidiuretic hormone; → = stimulatory (positive) influence; - - - ‖ = inhibitory (negative) influence.

B. **Feedback loops in the regulation of arterial blood pressure** (Fig. 2)

Because of their number and complexity, no attempt is made here to cover all feedback and reflex mechanisms. Rather, an overview of the clinically most relevant ones is presented. For further information, the reader is referred to appropriate reviews listed at the end of this chapter.

1. **Rapid responses and reflexes** (seconds)

   a. A **rise** in arterial blood pressure causes the baroreceptor system to respond by inhibiting sympathetic output and stimulating parasympathetic output (via the vagus nerve) from the central vasomotor center of the brainstem. This results in

      i. Decreased sympathetic outflow to arterioles (decreasing peripheral resistance)

      ii. Decreased sympathetic outflow to veins (decreasing cardiac filling pressure)

      iii. Decreased sympathetic tone to the heart (slowing heart rate and reducing contractility)

      iv. Increased parasympathetic tone to the heart (slowing heart rate and reducing contractility

      v. Little change in antidiuretic hormone (ADH) secretion

         (a) Baroreceptors tonically inhibit ADH secretion normally

         (b) During hypotension this tone decreases, leading to increased release of ADH (vasopressin)

(c) In cases of severe hypotension, the vasoconstrictor action of ADH becomes important (and rapid)

(d) The antidiuretic effect of ADH is a component of the slower-acting responses and is not important in the rapid feedback-mechanisms (see below)

b. Although several pathways are activated in the baroreceptor arc, each limb (represented in Fig. 2 by separate connections via the vagus and sympathetic fibers) is capable of being activated separately under certain circumstances

c. **Chemoreceptors** also act at the vasomotor center but respond not only to arterial pressure but also to oxygen tension and carbon dioxide tension (in opposite directions). A **drop** in arterial pressure, a drop in oxygen tension, or a rise in carbon dioxide tension results in

  i. **Increased sympathetic outflow** to skeletal arterioles
  ii. **Increased vagal tone**, leading to slowing of heart rate

d. The **central nervous system** (CNS, including supratentorial connections) senses ischemia or a rise in carbon dioxide in much the same way as the chemoreceptors

2. **Intermediate-acting responses** (minutes to hours)

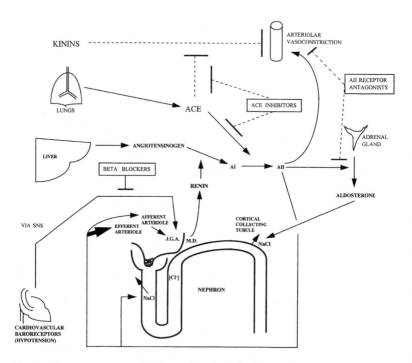

FIGURE 3. The renin-angiotensin system in the control of blood pressure. AI = angiotensin I; AII = angiotensin II; J.G.A. = juxtaglomerular apparatus; M.D. = macula densa; [Cl⁻] = luminal chloride concentration; S.N.S. = sympathetic nervous system; → = positive influence; - - - ‖ = negative influence. ACE = angiotensin-converting enzyme.

a. **Renin-angiotensin system** (RAS) (Fig. 3): both systemic and local systems are known to function; maladaptive responses to angiotensin II (AII),[8,9] which are long-term, are not shown

  i. Systemic RAS (Fig. 3)

    (a) Renin secretion from juxtaglomerular apparatus is stimulated by

      (i) Afferent arteriole baroreceptor when pressure drops

      (ii) Macula densa mechanism: renin secretion varies inversely with the chloride concentration reaching the thick ascending loop of Henle[1]

    (b) Increased activity of renal sympathetic nerves also increases renin release and often accompanies increased sympathetic outflow from other feedback loops, including aortic baroreceptors

    (c) Renin acts by converting angiotensinogen (A) (synthesized in the liver but also locally) to angiotensin I (AI)

    (d) Angiotensin I (AI) is converted to AII by angiotensin converting enzyme (ACE), produced in the lung (and locally)

    (e) ACE is also a kininase and reduces the concentration of vasodilatory kinins

    (f) AII has at least three effects

      (i) It is a potent vasoconstrictor (acting over minutes to hours)

      (ii) It causes the adrenal gland to produce aldosterone over the next several hours; aldosterone leads to volume expansion due to sodium retention

      (iii) It directly increases proximal NaCl absorption

  ii. Local RAS (Fig. 4)

    (a) Found in

      (i) Vasculature   (iii) Brain   (v) Adrenal

      (ii) Heart   (iv) Kidney   (vi) Testes

    (b) With the possible exception of renin, which in some cases may be taken up by tissues from the blood stream, local RASs may function independently of the systemic RAS

    (c) It is unclear if the local RAS is important in immediate, intermediate, or long-acting responses in the cardiovascular system

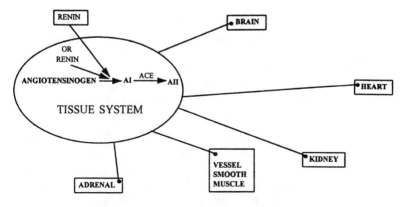

FIGURE 4. The tissue renin-angiotensin systems.

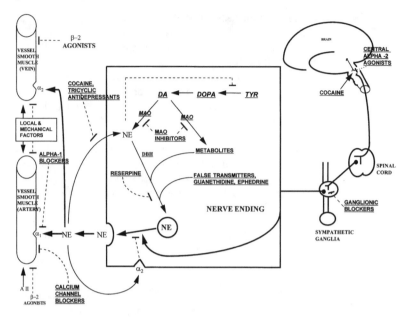

FIGURE 5. Neuropharmacologic interactions in the treatment of hypertension. AII = angiotensin II; NE = norepinephrine; TYR = tyrosine; DOPA = dihydroxyphenylalanine; DA = dopamine; MAO = monoamine oxidase; DBH = dopamine β-hydroxylase; α_1 = α_1-receptors; α_2 = α_2-receptors. → = stimulatory (positive) influence; - - - ‖ = inhibitory (negative) influence.

    b. **Antidiuretic hormone** (ADH) (Fig. 2)
        i. ADH secretion **increases in response to decreased blood volume** via a decrease in inhibitory tone from the **baroreceptors** to the hypothalamus
        ii. A **rise in arterial pressure causes a decrease in secretion of ADH** related to increased baroreceptor activity, which inhibits hypothalamic ADH-releasing neurons
        iii. Although increased secretion occurs in response to both increasing plasma osmolality and reduced intravascular volume, the response to rising osmolality is more immediate, whereas the response to reduced blood pressure (volume) is of greater magnitude
        iv. ADH works by causing water conservation at the distal collecting duct of the nephron. This alone, without salt conservation, is a relatively inefficient mechanism of increasing intravascular volume because conserved water is distributed among total body water and only a small portion is intravascular
        v. ADH levels in the sitting position have been found to be 2- to 3-fold higher in African-Americans vs. Caucasians[2]; moreover, calcium antagonists have been shown to blunt the blood pressure elevating effects of ADH in this population[3]
    c. **Capillary filtration** (not shown): at higher arterial pressures, some fluid transudes across capillaries and into the interstitial space, reducing blood volume

3. **Late-acting mechanisms** (days to weeks): although these mechanisms take longer to activate, their long-term efficiency (gain) is greater than that of the shorter-acting systems
   a. **Renal-body fluid system** (hours to days)
      i. A rise in arterial pressure leads to increased salt and water excretion directly (pressure diuresis)
      ii. ADH, in addition to acting in the immediate response to severe hypotension as a pressor and in the intermediate response to conserve blood volume, continues water conservation as long as the stimulus exists and therefore is also a late-acting response
C. **Receptors mediating the control of blood pressure** (Table 1)
   1. **Alpha-1 receptors:** pressure is lowered by antagonism of the peripheral postsynaptic receptor on the **arterioles**
   2. **Alpha-2 receptors**
      a. CNS synapse

TABLE I. Adrenergic Receptors in the Modulation of Arterial Blood Pressure

Receptors	Agonist Actions	Agonists	Antagonists
Alpha-1	Vasoconstriction*	Norepinephrine > > dopamine > dolbutamine	Prazosin, labetalol
Alpha-2, central effect	Vasodilation	Clonidine, norepinephrine	
Alpha-2, peripheral effect	Venoconstriction	Clonidine, norepinephrine	
Alpha-1 and alpha-2	Net vasoconstriction; reflex decreased cardiac output	Ergot, midodrine, norepinephrine > epinephrine	Phentolamine, Phenoxybenzamine
Beta-1	Increased cardiac output, lipolysis, increased renin	Epinephrine, norepinephrine, low-dose dopamine, dobutamine*	Atenolol, metoprolol
Beta-2	Vasodilation,[†] bronchodilation	Albuterol, epinephrine > > norepinephrine	
Beta-1 and beta-2	Net increased cardiac output	Epinephrine, isoproterenol	Propranolol, pindolol
Alpha-1 and beta-1	Vasoconstriction and increased cardiac output	Epinephrine, high-dose dopamine	Labetalol
Parasympathetic	Decreased cardiac output, decreased heart rate	Acetylcholine	Atropine
V_1	Increased peripheral resistance	Arginine vasopressin	Selective V_1 receptor antagonists (not commercially available) or calcium antagonists

* Predominantly arteriolar.
[†] Without chronotropic effects (unlike dopamine and isoproterenol).

      i. **Stimulation is inhibitory** to the vasomotor output to arterioles, thereby **decreasing** peripheral neuron discharges and lowering peripheral resistance

      ii. Slowing of beta-1 output also may occur through the same mechanism at the heart

  b. Primary constrictor receptor on veins

      i. Stimulation increases venous return

      ii. The potential of increased venous return to cause increased cardiac output, and therefore higher pressure, is more than offset by arteriolar and cardiac effects due to baroreflexes, in patients with an intact peripheral sympathetic nervous system

3. **Beta-1 receptors**

  a. Heart

      i. Stimulation results in increased heart rate

      ii. Stimulation results in increased force of contraction

  b. Kidney: stimulation results in increased renin output (see Fig. 3)

4. **Beta-2 receptors**

  a. Arterioles: stimulation results in relaxation

  b. Bronchioles: stimulation results in relaxation

D. **Neurotransmitters**

  1. **Epinephrine** (alpha-1, alpha-2 and beta-1, beta-2)

    a. Increase in heart rate

    b. No change or drop in blood pressure

  2. **Norepinephrine** (alpha-1 and alpha-2 only): hypertension without change in heart rate

E. **Neurochemical interactions in the action of neuropharmacologic agents and blood vessel diameter** (see Fig. 5)

  1. A blood pressure center within the brainstem is influenced by many forces, including baroreceptor feedback and supratentorial connections.

    a. **Stimulation of central alpha-2 receptors** inhibits alpha-1 and beta-1 output from the brainstem

  2. Neurons, projecting from the brainstem, synapse in the cord and those neurons, in turn, terminate in the sympathetic ganglia.

    a. **Ganglionic blockers** function at the sympathetic ganglia to block impulses there

  3. Electrical impulses cause release of norepinephrine stored in granules

    a. **Guanethidine** acts by replacing norephinephrine by incorporation into granules, thereby depleting stores of norepinephrine

    b. **Reserpine** blocks incorporation of neurotransmitter (norepinephrine) into granules

  4. After release from the presynaptic cell, norepinephrine molecules attach to alpha receptors on effector cells

    a. **Peripheral alpha-1** and **nonselective alpha blockers** prevent this attachment

  5. After norepinephrine attaches to the effector alpha-1 receptor, a calcium channel activates the change in length of the muscle fibers.

    a. The uptake of calcium is blocked by calcium channel blockers (see below and chapter 4)

6. On reaching the extracellular cleft, norepinephrine is removed by reuptake into the presynaptic cell and generalized metabolism via the blood stream.
   a. Reuptake is blocked by **tricyclic antidepressants**
7. Norepinephrine also feeds back to alpha-2 receptors on the presynaptic nerve ending to lessen norepinephrine release.
   a. This action is blocked by **nonspecific alpha blockers** and **alpha-2 blockers**

II. Mechanisms of Antihypertensive drugs

A. Central agents (alpha-2 agonists)

1. **Clonidine**
   a. By stimulating *central* alpha-2 receptors, *reduces* central sympathetic outflow to the *peripheral* beta-1 receptors and *peripheral* alpha-1 receptors; without intact nervous system, peripheral alpha-2 stimulation may predominate, leading to venoconstriction
      i. Decreased cardiac output
      ii. Relative reduction in tendency of heart rate to rise
      iii. Baroreceptor reflexes are preserved
      iv. Little change in peripheral resistance
   b. Acts directly on venous alpha-2 receptors to cause venoconstriction
2. **Methyldopa**
   a. Decreases sympathetic outflow to the alpha-1 receptors of the arterioles, thereby reducing peripheral resistance with little (but some) effect on the heart. Some antinatriuretic effect occurs (probably due to some reduction in renal vascular resistance)
   b. Baroreceptor arc impaired because of effect on arterioles

B. "Direct" vasodilators (hydralazine, diazoxide, minoxidil)

1. Arteriolar effects only; most work by opening cellular potassium channels (e.g., minoxidil)
2. No direct cardiac effects; therefore, when used alone, direct vasodilators lead to reflex increases in heart rate and force of contraction
3. Simultaneous use of beta blockers and diuretics required in most cases

C. Inhibitors of vasoconstriction

1. **Calcium channel blockers**
   a. Cause arteriolar without venous dilation (more precisely, attenuate vasoconstriction)
   b. At least 4 classes of calcium channel blockers available in U.S.
      i. L-channel blockers: the three different classes work on different sites within the L channel and hence produce different effects in the kidney, heart, and vasculature
         (a) Benzothiazepines (diltiazem is only drug in this class available in U.S.)
         (b) Phenylalkylamines (verapamil is only drug in this class available in U.S.)
         (c) Dihydropyridines
            (i) Nifedipine
            (ii) Isradipine
            (iii) Amlodipine
            (iv) Felodipine
            (v) Nisoldipine

   (vi) Nimodipine (used for treatment of cerebral vasospasm accompanying subarachnoid hemorrhage; not used for treatment of hypertension)

  ii. Diarylaminopropylene ethers (bepridil, used for angina pectoris refractory to most other measures; not used for treatment of hypertension without refractory angina)

 c. Calcium channel blockers of different classes differ in their effects

  i. Verapamil and diltiazem blunt increases in heart rate in response to exercise and have both negative inotropic and negative chronotropic effects (verapamil > diltiazem); most dihydropyridines do not have major cardiodepressant effects because the long-acting agents slightly increase sympathetic nervous system tone; short-acting agents even more so

  ii. In general, dihydropyridines lead to increases in heart rate and do not blunt the increase in heart rate response to exercise; among dihydropyridines the following differences have been noted

   (a) Nicardipine may have greater antianginal effect and less dizziness than nifedipine[4]

   (b) Amlodipine also seems to produce both coronary and peripheral vasodilation but with less reflex tachycardia possibly because of its long half-life[5,6]

   (c) Isradipine has a vasodilator effect similar to that of nifedipine, but also has a direct negative chronotropic effect on SA node and thus leads to little or no increase in heart rate

 d. Relative impairment of cardiac conduction prevents reflex tachycardia with verapamil and diltiazem

 e. Calcium channel blockers have a slight transient natriuretic effect; therefore, total body sodium retention does not occur within the first week of use

 f. Because arterioles are preferentially affected, transcapillary pressure increases, which may lead to local dependent edema, especially without a negative inotropic effect

  i. This effect is most prominent with the dihydropyridine calcium channel blockers

  ii. *ACE inhibitors are the treatment of choice for this edema*

 g. Drugs with greater cardiac depressant effects result in lesser peripheral edema, but greater tendency for decrease in cardiac conduction and reduction in cardiac output; drugs with less cardiodepressant effects lead to an increase in cardiac output and more peripheral edema

 h. All calcium channel blockers act primarily to dilate afferent and not efferent arterioles of the glomeruli; other differential effects of these agents on the kidney are listed in Table 2

  i. Dihydropyridine calcium channel blockers eliminate renal autoregulation; therefore, renal protection with dihydropyridines may require systolic blood pressure under 110 mmHg[6,7]

  ii. Nondihydropyridines only partially inhibit renal autoregulation[6]

2. **Alpha blockers**

 a. Nonselective alpha blockers

TABLE 2. Summary of Intrarenal Hemodynamic and Morphologic Effects of Antihypertensive Drug Classes in Animal Models of Diabetes

Effects	ACEIs/ARBs	Calcium Channel Blockers		α-Blockers	Diuretics	β-Blockers
		DHP	NDHP			
Hemodynamics						
P_{GC}	↓	→	→	→	→	→
R_A (tone)	↑	↑↑	↑	↑↑	→	→↓
R_e (tone)	↓	→	→↓	→	↑	→
ΔP	→↓	→	→↓	→	→	→
Autoregulation	→	↓↓	→	→	↓*	→
Glomerular permeability	↓	→↑	↓	→	?	?
Morphology						
Vv	↓	→	↓	→	?	?
Glomerulosclerosis	↓↓	→	↓	→	→	↓
Matrix proteins	↓↓	→	→	?	?	?

Vv = mesangial matrix expansion, P_{GC} = intraglomerular pressure, → = no effect, ↑ = increase, ↓ = decrease, ? = not established, * = loop diuretics only, R_A = afferent arteriolar tone, R_e = efferent arteriolar tone, ACEI = ACE inhibitors, ARBs = angiotensin II receptor blockers, ΔP = transcapillary pressure.

    i. Because they block both the postsynaptic receptor site and the presynaptic feedback site, catecholamine build-up within certain cells may lead to tachycardia due to release of catecholamines into the circulation with unopposed beta stimulation of the heart (tachycardia) and tachyphylaxis at other sites including the arterioles

    ii. Nonselective inhibition of alpha receptors in the gut leads to nausea, vomiting, and diarrhea

  b. Selective alpha-1 blockers

    i. Block action of norepinephrine at arteriolar receptors

    ii. Do not interfere with feedback of norepinephrine; therefore, no catecholamine build-up occurs

D. **Beta blockers**

  1. Nonselective beta blockers without intrinsic sympathomimetic activity (ISA)

    a. Central side effects (see appendices V and VII)

    b. Antagonize sympathetic stimulation of renin secretion (see Fig. 3)

    c. Reduce cardiac output and heart rate

  2. Nonselective beta blockers with ISA

    a. Intrinsic beta-1 agonist activity prevents direct cardiac effects

    b. Noncardiac beta-2 stimulation leads to vasodilation

    c. "Blockade" occurs mainly in response to stimuli

  3. Beta-1 selective agents

    a. Have more effect on cardiac output and renin

    b. Have less effect on peripheral resistance and bronchi

  4. Beta-1 selective blockers with ISA

    a. Block beta-1 receptors at the heart and yet apparently have beta-2 agonist activity

E. **Diuretics**

  1. Cause sodium loss

  2. Cause some degree of vasodilation

F. **Angiotensin-converting enzyme inhibitors**
   1. Inhibit renin-mediated AII production
   2. Have additional effects independent of systemic renin-angiotensin axis which are poorly understood but may include
      a. Vasodilation dependent on increased levels of kinins because converting enzyme is also a kininase[8]
      b. Vasodilation due to increase in certain prostaglandins
   3. In patients with relatively low plasma renin levels, ACE inhibition may work through inhibition of **local** renin-angiotensin systems in vascular endothelium and possibly even the brain[8,9]

G. **Angiotensin receptor antagonists** (AII blockers)
   1. Inhibit angiotensin II action at receptors. Currently available agents block only AT-1 but not AT-2 receptors
   2. Do not affect angiotensin-converting enzyme; therefore no change in kinin concentrations (angiotensin converting enzyme is a kininase; this may explain the occasionally lower potency of AII blockers as antihypertensives)
   3. Selectively inhibit the AT-1 receptors in the heart and blood vessels leading to regression of left ventricular hypertrophy vasodilation in animal models; they do not inhibit AT-2 receptors which may contribute to this and other changes[10–12]

H. Influence of various drugs on intrarenal hemodynamics and morphology (see Table 2)
   1. ACE inhibitors reduce glomerular transcapillary pressure by reducing efferent arteriolar tone to a greater extent than other agents; they also reduce mesangial expansion
   2. Nondihydropyridine calcium channel blockers seem to be the only other agents that may reduce efferent arteriolar tone and reduce mesangial expansion

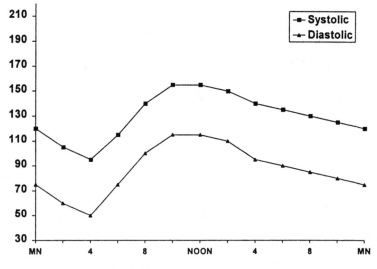

FIGURE 6. Circadian variation in blood pressure.

    3. The above two classes are the only ones shown to reduce glomerulosclerosis in experimental animals

III. **Circadian Variation of Blood Pressure**

  A. **Normal circadian rhythms**

    1. In most normal patients, blood pressure nadirs during the night and peaks shortly after rising in the morning (Fig. 6)

    2. This rise and fall in blood pressure correlates with many other factors

      a. Catecholamine levels
      b. Cortisol levels
      c. Heart rate
      d. Pulse-pressure product
      e. Increase in platelet adhesiveness
      f. Plasma renin activity
      g. Plasma aldosterone
      h. Arterial compliance
      i. Blood viscosity

    3. Most people's blood pressure peaks about 3 hours after awakening (range 6:00 a.m. to 12:00 noon)

    4. Some patients may have second peak
      a. Usually around 6:00–9:00 p.m.
      b. Usually smaller rise than upon awakening

  B. **In some patients with clinical illnesses,** different pattern may be seen:

    1. For first month after acute myocardial infarction, patients have been reported to have largest peaks in ischemia (which usually correlate with blood pressure) between 6:00 p.m. and 12:00 a.m.

    2. In many other states, evening and morning peaks may be equal; in some cases, the peak may occur at night ("nondippers")[13–15]; this pattern has been reported in **some** patients with the following:
      a. Diabetes mellitus
      b. Congestive heart failure
      c. Female sex
      d. Elderly patients
      e. Patients with autonomic neuropathy
      f. Smokers
      g. Sleep apnea syndrome
      h. Renal transplant recipients (independent of drug effects)[15]
      i. Chronic renal failure

    3. Some studies suggest that "nondippers" may have worse prognosis than "dippers"[16,17]
      a. The definitions of "nondipping" are not established; one recent study suggested a definition of nocturnal pressure **higher** than daytime pressure; in reality this is **reversal** of what has been traditionally considered the normal diurnal variation of pressure[18]
      b. How diurnal variations of blood pressure should influence therapy is also unclear
        i. One study found that excessive dipping at night in patients treated with antihypertensive drugs was associated with an increased risk of stroke[19] in patients with a prior history of cerebrovascular disease
        ii. Another study showed that higher nocturnal blood pressure was associated with increased microalbuminuria in non–insulin-dependent diabetics[20]
        iii. "Nondippers" have a higher incidence of both microalbuminuria and left ventricular hypertrophy[19,20]

REFERENCES

1. Lorenz JN, Greenberg SG, Briggs JP: The macula densa mechanism for control of renin secretion. Semin Nephrol 1993;13:531–542.
2. Bakris GL, Bursztyn M, Gavras I, et al: Role of vasopressin in essential hypertension: Racial differences. J Hypertens 1997;15:545–550.
3. Bakris GL, Kusmirek SL, Smith AC: Calcium antagonism abolishes the antipressor action of vasopressin (V_1) receptor antagonism. Am J Hypertens 1997;10:1153–1158.
4. De Wood MA, Wolbach RA: Randomized double-blind comparison of side effects of nicardipine and nifedipine in angina pectoris. The nicardipine investigators group. Am Heart J 1990;119:468–478.
5. Van Zwieten PA, Pfaffendorf M: Similarities and differences between calcium antagonists: Pharmacological aspects. J Hypertens 1993;11S:S3–S11.
6. Tarif N, Bakris GL: Preservation of renal function: The spectrum of effects by calcium channel blockers. Nephrol Dial Transplant 1997;12:2244–2250.
7. Griffin KA, Picken MM, Bidani AK: Deleterious effects on calcium channel blockade on pressure transmission and glomerular injury in rat remnant kidneys. J Clin Invest 1995;96:798–800.
8. Williams GH: Converting enzyme inhibitors in the treatment of hypertension. N Engl J Med 1988;319:1517–1525.
9. Redgrave J, Rabinowe S, Hollenberg NK, Williams GH: Correction of abnormal renal blood flow response to angiotensin II by converting enzyme inhibition in essential hypertension. J Clin Invest 1985;75:1285–1290.
10. Johnston CI: Renin-angiotensin system: A dual tissue and hormonal system for cardiovascular control. J Hypertens 1992;10(Suppl 7):S13.
11. Levy BI, Benessiano J, Henrion D, et al: Chronic blockade of AT2-subtype receptors prevents the effect of angiotensin II on the rat vascular structure. J Clin Invest 1996;98:418.
12. Stoll M, Steckelingd UM, et al: The angiotensin AT-2 receptor mediates inhibition of cell proliferation in coronary endothelial cells. J Clin Invest 1995;95:651.
13. Hjalmarson A, Gilpin EA, Nicod P, et al: Differing circadian patterns of symptom onset in subgroups of patients with acute myocardial infarction. Circulation 1989;80:267–275.
14. Hanson O, Johansson BW, Gullberg B: Circadian distribution of onset of acute myocardial infarction in subgroups from analysis of 10,791 patients treated in a single center. Am J Cardiol 1992;69:1003–1008.
15. Smolensky MH: Chronobiology and chronotherapeutics. Applications to cardiovascular medicine. Am J Hypertens 1996;9:11S–21S.
16. Verdecchia P, Schillaci G, Guerrieri M, et al: Circadian blood pressure changes and left ventricular hypertrophy in essential hypertension Circulation 1990;81:528–536.
17. Verdecchia P, Schillaci G, Gatteschi C, et al: Blunted nocturnal fall in blood pressure in hypertensive women with future cardiovascular morbid events. Circulation 1993;88(3):986–992.
18. Staessen JA, Bieniaszewski L, O'Brien E, et al: Nocturnal blood pressure fall on ambulatory monitoring in a large international database. Hypertension 1997;29(1 Pt 1):30–39.
19. Nakamura P, Oita J, Yamaguchi T: Nocturnal blood pressure dip in stroke survivors. Stroke 1995;26:1373–1378.
20. Mitchell TH, Nolan B, Henry M, et al: Microalbuminuria in patients with non-insulin-dependent diabetes mellitus relates to nocturnal systolic blood pressure. Am J Med 1997;102:531–535.

CHAPTER 2

Definitions, Epidemiology, Natural History, and Prognosis

I. **Types of Hypertension**
  A. **Essential hypertension**
    1. Defined as persistent elevation of arterial pressure that results from dys-regulation of normal homeostatic control mechanisms in the absence of detectable known secondary cause
    2. Definitions of **stages of hypertension** reflecting severity, according to the Joint National Committee on Detection, Evaluation and Treatment of High Blood Pressure (JNC VI) guidelines,[1] are presented in Table 3. Previous stages III and IV have been combined

TABLE 3.   Stages of Hypertension (JNC VI)*

Category	Systolic (mmHg) **or** Diastolic (mmHg)	
Optimal	< 120	< 80
Normal	< 130	< 85
High normal (borderline)	130–139	85–89
Stage I (mild)	140–159	90–99
Stage II (moderate)	160–179	100–109
Stage III (severe)	≥ 180	≥ 110

* The stage is defined by the **higher** of the systolic or diastolic pressure.

    3. JNC VI has suggested classifying hypertension not only on the basis of arterial blood pressure but also by risk[1] and then basing treatment on stratification, taking into account both pressure and risk (Table 4)
  B. **Pseudohypertension**
    1. Readings taken with blood pressure cuff are elevated and do not reflect the true blood pressure measured directly by intraarterial cannula
    2. Caused by relatively incompressible peripheral vessels due to calcific atherosclerosis
    3. Hypertensive end-organ damage is absent
    4. May be detected in some patients via Osler's maneuver (see Physical examination, Chapter 3)

TABLE 4.   Classification of Risk Factors Associated with Increased Morbidity and Mortality in Hypertensive Patients

Group A	Group B	Group C
≤ 159 Systolic or ≤ 99 diastolic (stage I or less)	≥ 140 Systolic or ≥ 90 diastolic (stage I or more)	≥ 130 Systolic or ≥ 85 diastolic (high normal or more)
and	**and**	**and**
No risk factors*	≥ 1 Risk factor*	Manifest azotemia, congestive heart failure, diabetes mellitus, or other cardiovascular disease
Treatment:	Treatment:	Treatment:
Vigorous nondrug therapy for up to 1 year	Consider aggressive therapy; lower pressure to ≤ 139/84	Aggressive therapy; for patients with congestive heart failure, diabetes mellitus, or azotemia, to optimal levels as tolerated (≤ 120/80)

Modified from JNC VI.[1]
* See pages 19 and 31.

C. **Systolic hypertension**
1. Proven benefit in treating, mainly in stroke prevention[2]
2. Shows greater correlation with end-stage renal disease than diastolic hypertension[3]

D. **Reactive hypertension:** secondary to acute event
1. In many cases, studies indicate that more harm than good may come from treatment
   a. Drug withdrawal
   b. Psychosis
   c. Seizures
   d. Stroke
   e. Hypertension due to pain
   f. Hypertension due to hypoxemia
   g. Hypertension due to ischemia
2. Treatment of reactive hypertension during or immediately following stroke is **generally not recommended**, and no studies in animals or humans suggest that reactive hypertension following stroke should be treated[4]
   a. Elevated blood pressure following stroke decreases in patients given antihypertensives at rate comparable to rate that it decreases spontaneously[5,6]
   b. Treated patients do not have improvement in cerebral blood flow and in fact may have a **decrease** in cerebral blood flow to areas surrounding the infarction, causing extension of infarct size[7]
   c. Serious complications of such treatment are reported[8]
   d. Consensus favors withholding aggressive drug therapy[3,5–7,9]
   e. Level of elevation at which treatment should be considered (if any) is debated, because no data show that treating even very high pressures is beneficial[4–6,8,9]
   f. In **subarachnoid hemorrhage**, nimodipine has shown value in reducing cerebral vasospasm responsible for posthemorrhagic ischemia, but treatment is **not** aimed at blood pressure control and reversal of ischemia does not correlate with blood pressure reduction;[10–13] reduction of blood pressure in such patients is potentially risky, particularly if the patient has hydrocephalus, intracranial hemorrhage, or evidence of vasospasm[4]

E. **"White-coat" hypertension and labile hypertension**
1. The patient's blood pressure is elevated mainly in the office ("white-coat" hypertension) or alternates between normal and elevated (labile hypertension)
2. Although this disorder was suspected to be completely benign, available data suggest that risk may be intermediate between normal and persistent (sustained) hypertension[14]
3. Echocardiography may have role in deciding if treatment is warranted

F. **Accelerated hypertension:** end-organ damage without papilledema or medical emergency
1. Advancing renal insufficiency
2. Funduscopic hemorrhages without papilledema

G. **Malignant hypertension:** one or more of the following
1. Papilledema and/or
2. Pulmonary edema and/or
3. Neurologic findings and/or
4. Hypertension-induced angina

H. **Secondary hypertension:** defined as persistent hypertension due to second, underlying disorder other than essential hypertension (see Chapters 3 and 6, Appendices I–IV)

I. **Resistant hypertension** is defined as follows[1]
1. Blood pressure > 140/90 mmHg while patient is taking 3 or more drugs in near-maximal doses, one of which is a diuretic
2. In isolated systolic hypertension, 160 mmHg despite similar regimen

II. **Basic Statistics**
A. Incidence: approximately 20% of general adult population[15]
B. Frequency of diagnosis (1991–1994): about 10% of patients with hypertension are unaware of their diagnosis, a marked improvement from prior statistics[1]
C. Frequency of treatment, control,[15] and complications
1. About 54% are under treatment
2. Only 27.4% of patients have reached levels of < 140/90 mmHg
3. Despite the slight improvement in proportion of treated patients, incidence of stroke and congestive heart failure has increased.[1] Moreover, progression to end-stage renal disease continues to increase.[1]
D. Incidence by type (adults)
1. Essential: 90–92%
2. Renal: < 3%
   a. Parenchymal: $\frac{2}{3}$
   b. Renovascular: $\frac{1}{3}$
3. Birth control pill usage: < 3%
4. Primary aldosteronism: 0.3–1%
5. Cushing's syndrome: < 0.1%
6. Pheochromocytoma: < 0.1%
7. Miscellaneous: 0.2%

III. **Confounding Variables in Essential Hypertension**
A. Genetics: strong family history in most patients
B. Environmental factors
1. Salt sensitivity in about 60% of essential hypertension (especially diabetics, African-Americans, and others)
2. Obesity
C. Gender
1. Prevalence[15]
   a. More common in men than women until age 60
   b. In African-American and Hispanic people older than 60, more common in women
   c. In Caucasians over 80, 14% higher incidence in women, especially for systolic hypertension
2. Left ventricular hypertrophy is more likely to result from isolated systolic hypertension in women than men[16]
3. Strokes: more frequently hypertension-related in women than men[17]
4. Congestive heart failure: more likely to result from hypertension in women[20]
5. Elderly women with isolated systolic hypertension are at least as likely as men to benefit from treatment[18]
6. Drug side effects

       a. Although sexual dysfunction has not been reported as often in women as in men, available studies may not have detected such dysfunction because of study design[19]

       b. ACE inhibitor–induced cough much more common in women[20,21]

   7. African-American women are more likely to have hypertension than African-American men and benefit more from treatment than Caucasian women, regardless of age[22]

   8. Reactive ("white-coat") hypertension: more common in women[23,24]

IV. Natural History and Consequences

  A. Increased risk of atherosclerosis

  B. If untreated, increases in severity

  C. Even if mild, yet left untreated, leads to high incidence of end-organ damage

V. Prognosis

  A. Treatment of even mild hypertension is associated with decrease in incidence of stroke[25,26]

  B. Factors associated with higher morbidity and/or mortality

    1. African-American race

    2. Onset in youth

    3. Consistently higher pressure (> 160/100 mmHg)

    4. Smoking

    5. Dyslipidemia

    6. Obesity

    7. Diabetes mellitus (doubles risk)

    8. Male gender

    9. Evidence of end-organ damage, *left ventricular hypertrophy by electrocardiographic criteria, elevated serum creatinine ≥ 1.4 mg/dl*

   10. Hyperinsulinemia (even without frank diabetes)

   11. Syndrome X

     a. Coronary artery disease

     b. Dyslipidemia

     c. Hypertension

     d. Hyperinsulinemia

     e. Hyperuricemia

  C. Stress and hypertension

    1. Stress may transiently elevate blood pressure

    2. Such elevations have **not** been shown to cause morbidity or lead to sustained hypertension[27]

  D. Hypertension and end-stage renal disease

    1. In 1997, 34% of end-stage renal disease was attributed to hypertension[28] (second only to diabetic nephropathy)

    2. In MRFIT trials, although both systolic and diastolic hypertension correlated with development of end-stage renal disease, **systolic hypertension seemed to show a higher correlation with development of end-stage renal disease.**[29] Moreover, in retrospective studies systolic blood pressure correlates more strongly with development of renal disease than diastolic blood pressure

    3. Multiple studies show that all stages of hypertension can lead to renal failure, although progression to end-stage renal disease is seen primarily in patients with stages II and III hypertension[30]

4. Available data suggest direct correlation between azotemia and rise in blood pressure of 20 mmHg, even when still within the "normal" range.[31] This finding suggests that, at least in some patients, rise in pressure from baseline, regardless of how low it may be in the beginning, also may be risk factor

5. African-Americans are at particularly high risk for cardiorenal problems
   a. Develop hypertension earlier than Caucasians
   b. Develop more severe hypertension than Caucasians
   c. Develop end-stage renal disease much more frequently than Caucasians, especially those with higher systolic blood pressures[32]

6. Diabetic nephropathy progression
   a. Dramatically accelerated by hypertension
   b. Dramatically slowed by treatment of hypertension
      i. Particularly with agents that inhibit the renin-angiotensin system such as ACE inhibitors
      ii. Angiotensin receptor blockers appear to be as effective in preventing diabetic renal disease as ACE inhibitors in animal models; however, human clinical trial data are pending[33–39]
      iii. Goals of treatment to lower blood pressure to < 130/85 mmHg (see Chapter 4, pages 57–58)

7. Progression of hypertensive nephrosclerosis seems to slow dramatically when blood pressure is below 130/85[33–39]

8. Hypertensive patients with underlying renal disease, regardless of cause, seem to benefit dramatically from blood pressure control and preferentially from ACE inhibitors[34–39]

REFERENCES

1. Sixth Report of the Joint National Committee on Detection, Evaluation, and Treatment of High Blood Pressure (JNC-VI). Arch Intern Med 1997;157:2413–2445.
2. SHEP Cooperative Research Group: Prevention of stroke by antihypertensive drug therapy. JAMA 1991;265:3256–3264.
3. Perneger TV, Nieto FJ, Whelton PK, et al: A prospective study of blood pressure and serum creatinine. Results form the "Clue" study and the ARIC study. JAMA 1993;269:488–493.
4. Powers WJ: Acute hypertension after stroke: The scientific basis for treatment decisions. Neurology 1993;43:461–467.
5. Britton M, Carlson A, de Faire U: Blood pressure course with acute stroke and matched controls. Stroke 1986;17:861–864.
6. Lisk DR, Grotta JC, Lamki LM, et al: Should hypertension be treated after acute stroke? A randomized controlled trial using spectral photon emission computerized tomography. Arch Neurol 1993;50:855–862.
7. Meyer JS, Shimazu K, Fukuuchi Y, et al: Impaired neurogenic cerebrovascular control and dysautoregulation after stroke. Stroke 1973;4:169–186.
8. Britton M, de Faire U, Helmers C: Hazards of therapy for excessive hypertension in acute stroke. Acta Med Scand 1980;207:253–257.
9. Calhoun DA, Oparil SO: Treatment of hypertensive crisis. N Engl J Med 1990;323:1177–1183.
10. Allen GS, Ahn HS, Preziosi TJ, et al: Cerebral arterial spasm: A controlled trial of nimodipine in patients with subarachnoid hemorrhage. N Engl J Med 1983;308:619–624.
11. Petruk KC, West M, Mohr G, et al: Nimodipine treatment in poor grade aneurysm patients. J Neurosurg 1988;68:505–517.
12. Phillipon J, Grob R, Dagreou F, et al: Prevention of vasospasm in subarachnoid hemorrhage: A controlled study of nimodipine. Acta Neurochir (Wien) 1986;82:110–117.

13. Pickard JD, Murray GD, Illingworth R, et al: Effect of oral nimodipine on cerebral infarction and outcome after subarachnoid hemorrhage: British Aneurysm Nimodipine Trial. BMJ 1989;298:636–642.

14. Cardillo C, De Felice F, Campia U, Folli G: Psychophysiological reactivity in white coat hypertension. Hypertension 1993;21:836–844.

15. Burt VL, Whelton P, Roccella EJ, et al: Prevalence of hypertension in the US adult population. Results from the Third National Health and Nutrition Examination Survey (NHANES III) 1988–91. Hypertension 1995;25:305–313.

16. Krumholz HM, Larson M, Levy D: Sex differences in cardiac adaptation to isolated systolic hypertension. Am J Cardiol 1993;72:310–313.

17. Levy D, Larson MG, et al: The progression from hypertension to congestive heart failure. JAMA 1996;275:1557–1562.

18. Kostis JB, Davis BR, et al (SHEP Cooperative Research Group): Prevention of heart failure by antihypertensive drug treatment in older persons with isolated systolic hypertension. JAMA 1997;278:212–216.

19. Hayes SN, Taler SJ: Hypertension in women: Current understanding of gender differences. Mayo Clin Proc 1998;73:157–165.

20. Gibson GR: Enalapril-induced cough. Arch Intern Med 1989;149:2701–2703.

21. Os I, Bratland B, et al: Female preponderance for lisinopril-induced cough in hypertension. Am J Hypertens 1994;7:1012–1015.

22. Anastos K, Charney P, et al: Hypertension in women: What is really known? The Woman's Caucus, Working Group on Women's Health of the Society of General Internal Medicine. Ann Intern Med 1991;115:287–293.

23. Verdecchia P, Schillaci G, et al: White coat hypertension and white coat effect: Similarities and differences. Am J Hypertens 1992;5:1–7.

24. Diamond JA, Krakoff LR, et al: Comparison of ambulatory blood pressure and amounts of left ventricular hypertrophy in men versus women with similar levels of hypertensive clinic blood pressures. Am J Cardiol 1997;79:505–508.

25. Materson BJ, Reda RJ, Cushman WJ, et al: Single drug therapy for hypertension in men: A comparison of six antihypertensive agents with placebo. N Engl J Med 1993;328:914–921.

26. Neaton JD, Grim RH Jr, Prineas RJ, et al: Treatment of mild hypertension study: Final results. JAMA 1993;270:713–724.

27. Freeman ZS: Stress and hypertension—A critical review. Med J Aust 1990;153:621–625.

28. US Renal Data System: USRDS 1997 Annual Data Report. Bethesda, MD, National Institutes of Health, National Institute of Diabetes and Digestive and Kidney Diseases, 1997.

29. Klag MJ, Whelton PK, et al: Blood pressure and incidence of end-stage renal disease in men: A prospective study. Circulation 1994;18:941.

30. National High Blood Pressure Education Program Working Group: 1995 Update of the Working Group Reports on Chronic Renal Failure and Renovascular Hypertension. Arch Intern Med 1996;156:1938–1947.

31. Perneger TV, Niete FJ, et al: A prospective study of blood pressure and serum creatinine: Results from the Clue study and the ARIC study. JAMA 1993;269:488–493.

32. Perry HM, Miller JP, et al: Early predictors of 15-year end-stage renal disease in hypertensive patients. Hypertension 1995;25:587–594.

33. Bauer JH, Reams GP, Lai SM: Renal protective effect of strict blood pressure control with enalapril therapy. Arch Intern Med 1987;147:1387–1400.

34. Wee PM, De Michell AG, Epstein M: Effects of calcium antagonists on renal hemodynamics and progression of nondiabetic chronic renal disease. Arch Intern Med 1994;154:1185–1202.

35. Hannedouche T, Landais P, et al: Randomised controlled trial of enalapril and beta-blockers in non-diabetic chronic renal failure. BMJ 1994;309:833–837.

36. GISEN Study Group: Randomized placebo controlled trial of the effect of ramipiril on decline in glomerular filtration rate and risk of terminal renal failure in proteinuric nondiabetic nephropathy. Lancet 1997;349:1857–1863.

37. Maschio G, Alberti D, Hanin G, et al: Effect of the angiotensin-converting enzyme inhibitor benazapril on the progression of renal insufficiency. N Engl J Med 1996;334:939–945.

38. Tarif N, Bakris GL: Angiotensin II receptor blockade and progression of renal disease in non-diabetic patients. Kidney Int 1997;52(Suppl 63):S-67–S-70.
39. Bakris GL (ed): The renin-angiotensin system in diabetic nephropathy: From bench to bedside. Miner Electrolyte Metab 1998;24(6):361–438.

CHAPTER 3

Evaluation of the Patient with Hypertension

I. **Purposes of Evaluation**
   A. To uncover secondary causes of hypertension
   B. To establish a baseline and evaluate end-organ damage
   C. To determine additional risk factors
   D. To assess factors that may influence type of treatment
II. **Understanding the Causes of Secondary Hypertension**
   A. **Renal disorders:** most common causes of secondary hypertension
      1. **Renal parenchymal diseases**[1,2] (most common renal cause; 2–5% of hypertension)
         a. Examples
            i. Glomerular diseases
               (a) Idiopathic
               (b) Secondary (e.g., diabetic nephropathy, lupus erythematosus)
            ii. Tubulointerstitial diseases
               (a) Idiopathic
               (b) Secondary
            iii. Intrarenal vascular diseases
               (a) Scleroderma
               (b) Vasculitides
         b. Hypertension is earlier and more frequent with glomerular and vascular conditions than with tubulointerstitial diseases
         c. Majority of cases are volume (sodium)-dependent
         d. Most important and most frequent cause of secondary hypertension in children and adults
      2. **Renal artery stenosis**
         a. Major role of renin (at least in absence of sodium repletion)
         b. Cure rate by angioplasty
            i. 30% for nonostial atherosclerotic lesions
            ii. 50–90% for dysplasia
         c. Fibromuscular dysplasia is associated with
            i. Female gender
            ii. Neurofibromatosis
         d. Although incidence among African-Americans may be lower than among Caucasians, it is still substantial, and African-American hypertensives with features suggestive of renal artery stenosis should be investigated aggressively[3]
      3. **Urinary obstruction**
         a. Subtle at times
         b. Always consider, especially in
            i. Children
            ii. Diabetics
            iii. Elderly men
            iv. Labile hypertension
            v. Patients with recent pelvic surgery
         c. One of most important causes of labile hypertension
         d. May occur even with unilateral obstruction[27]
   B. **Endocrine and metabolic disorders**
      1. **Adrenal and adrenal-like entities**
         a. **Cushing's syndrome** (see Appendix I)

      i. Adrenal adenoma (or, rarely, carcinoma)

      ii. Hypothalamic/pituitary with adrenal hyperplasia

      iii. Ectopic secretion of adrenocorticotropic hormone (ACTH), especially from oat cell carcinoma

      iv. Drugs

b. **Primary hyperaldosteronism** (see Appendix II)

      i. High aldosterone usually with suppressed renin

      ii. Sodium-dependent

      iii. Hypokalemia usually a hallmark but this condition can be present with normal potassium values

      iv. Types

         (a) **Adenoma:** curable, often unilateral

         (b) **Hyperplasia:** usually bilateral, incurable, more orthostatic, less hypokalemic

         (c) **Glucocorticoid-suppressible hyperaldosteronism**[4]

            (i) Usually familial

            (ii) Onset usually before age 21 but can be in adulthood

            (iii) Autosomal dominant

            (iv) Usually not spontaneously hypokalemic but becomes hypokalemic with diuretics

            (v) Elevated 18-hydroxycortisol and 18-oxocortisol

            (vi) Diagnosis may be confirmed most easily through direct genetic analysis

            (vii) Should be suspected in patients with both (i) and (ii) above

c. **Gordon's syndrome** (hyperkalemic hypertensive syndrome; rare)[5]

      i. Hyperkalemia with distal (type I) renal tubular acidosis and hypertension

      ii. Clinical findings

         (a) Short stature

         (b) Muscle weakness

         (c) Intellectual impairment

         (d) Dental abnormalities

         (e) Impaired growth during childhood

         (f) Severe hypertension by third decade

      iii. Laboratory findings

         (a) Potassium typically > 6.5 mEq/L

         (b) Acidosis with inappropriately high urine pH (> 5.3)

         (c) Suppressed renin and elevated aldosterone during hyperkalemia

         (d) Serum aldosterone levels usually return toward normal after correction of serum potassium

      iv. Cause thought to be renal defect of sodium chloride hyperabsorption in distal tubule

      v. Dramatic improvement with salt restriction and/or thiazide diuretics

d. **Adrenogenital syndrome**

      i. Hypertensive forms rarely present with onset in adulthood

      ii. Elevated deoxycorticosterone (DOC) with suppressed plasma renin activity

         (a) 11-Hydroxylase deficiency (androgen excess)

         (b) 17-Hydroxylase deficiency (androgen and estrogen deficiency)

e. **Liddle's syndrome** (rare)[6-9]
    i. Presents with hypertension and hypokalemic alkalosis, often with muscle weakness, polydipsia, polyuria, and (in children) growth retardation and failure to thrive[10]
    ii. Both plasma renin activity and aldosterone are suppressed
    iii. Responds to triamterene or amiloride but not to spironolactone
f. **Apparent mineralocorticoid excess (AME) syndromes**[11] (see also Appendix II)
    i. Hypokalemia with suppressed renin and aldosterone, similar to Liddle syndrome
    ii. Defects caused by relative increase in ratio of cortisol to cortisone or excess of both
        (a) Deficiency of 11-beta hydroxysteroid dehydrogenase **(AME I)**
            (i) Congenital disease with severe hypertension
            (ii) Onset usually in childhood
            (iii) Rare condition with autosomal recessive inheritance
            (iv) Elevation of ratio of urinary metabolites of cortisol to those of cortisone (tetrahydrocortisol:tetrahydrocortisone ratio [THF:THE] > 1:1 is diagnostic)
            (v) Responds to spironolactone or dexamethasone, which suppresses ACTH
        (b) **AME II**
            (i) Recently some patients with normal THF:THE ratios have been noted and termed type II AME; such patients differ from patients with Liddle syndrome in that they respond to dexamethasone or spironolactone but not to triamterene
            (ii) Patients with either type I or type II AME may have reduced rate of A-ring reduction of cortisol, the step that transforms it into THF[13]
            (iii) Excessive cortisol accumulates and floods mineralocorticoid receptors with excessive cortisol
        (c) **Glycyrrhetinic acid**—found in black licorice (not available from U.S., but from Europe) and licorice-flavored foods, beverages, and tobacco, including certain cigars and chewing tobacco—by inhibiting 11-beta hydroxysteroid dehydrogenase, causes an acquired form of this syndrome
g. **Pheochromocytoma**[14] (see Appendix III)
    i. **50% of cases have sustained (nonparoxysmal) hypertension**
    ii. **Paroxysms of symptoms** often occur in patients with or without paroxysmal hypertension; **headache, sweating, and palpitations** are three most frequent symptoms, although often they do not occur together
    iii. **Other symptoms** in decreasing order of frequency
        (a) Pallor
        (b) Nervousness
        (c) Tremor
        (d) Nausea
        (e) Weakness
        (f) Abdominal pain
        (g) Dyspnea
        (h) Dizziness, heat intolerance, and/or flushing

iv. Most common paroxysms involve **hypertension, sweating, and tachycardia**. Attacks typically are brief and have acute onset (average attacks last 15 minutes)

v. Although face may be flushed, extremities are often pale

vi. **Precipitating factors** that may provoke attacks
   (a) Smoking
   (b) Induction of anesthesia
   (c) Ganglionic blockers
   (d) Hydralazine
   (e) Massage of tumor, bending, or voiding (especially with large or bladder tumors)

vii. Patient may present with hyperglycemia due to tumor and appear to have frequent "insulin reactions"

viii. Postural blood pressure drops are common

ix. Hypermetabolic states may occur with or without coexisting hyperthyroidism

x. **Associated entities**
   (a) Neurofibromatosis
   (b) von Hippel-Lindau syndrome
       (i) Renal cysts
       (ii) Cerebellar hemangioblastomas
       (iii) Pheochromocytomas
       (iv) Renal cell carcinomas
       (v) Retinal hemangioblastomas
       (vi) Angiomas and cysts of liver and pancreas
   (c) Tuberous sclerosis
       (i) Adenoma sebaceum (angiofibromas)
       (ii) Mental retardation
       (iii) Seizures
       (iv) Angioleiomyomas of kidney, liver, adrenal, pancreas
       (v) Pheochromocytomas
       (vi) Shagreen patches
       (vii) Ash-leaf "white spots"
   (d) Sturge-Weber syndrome
       (i) Trigeminal hemangiomas
       (ii) Seizures
       (iii) Mental retardation
   (e) Multiple endocrine neoplasia (MEN)
       (i) Type I (with neurofibromas, pituitary tumors, hyperparathyroidism, pancreatic islet cell tumors)
       (ii) Type IIa: similar to type I with medullary carcinoma of thyroid, usually no pancreatic tumors and:
           • IIa also have nonpituitary CNS tumors
           • IIb also have marfanoid features, retinal angiomas, mucosal neuromas, severe constipation but no CNS or pituitary tumors and no hyperparathyroidism
   (f) Familial pheochromocytoma (with or without islet cell tumors)

2. **Juxtaglomerular tumor and ectopic hyperreninism**
   a. Very rare

      b. Presents like hyperaldosteronism but with elevated plasma renin activity (PRA) and normal renal arteries

   3. **Acromegaly:** hypertension, atherosclerosis, and cardiac hypertrophy associated with

      a. Typical features of face and extremities
      b. Sweating
      c. Hypersomnolence
      d. Weight gain
      e. Goiter
      f. Carpal tunnel syndrome
      g. Visual field changes
      h. Hypertrichosis
      i. Enlarged furrowed tongue

   4. **Hypercalcemia**

      a. Particularly primary hyperparathyroidism
      b. May accompany pheochromocytoma

   5. **Birth control pill-induced hypertension**

      a. Associated with
         i. Age > 35 yr
         ii. Family history of hypertension
         iii. Obesity
         iv. Higher estrogen dosage formations
      b. Prognosis: 50% resolve within 6 months after drug stopped

   6. **Thyroid disorders**

      a. Hyperthyroidism: systolic hypertension
      b. Hypothyroidism: diastolic hypertension

C. **Coarctation of aorta**

   1. Physical findings (see Physical examination, page 31, III.B.)
   2. Rib notching and "3 sign" on chest radiograph

D. **Neurologic and neurovascular causes**

   1. Baroreflex failure syndrome

      a. Relatively rare entity that presents with symptoms, findings, and lab results similar to and sometimes not easily distinguished from pheochromocytoma

      b. Predisposing factors
         i. History of neck surgery
         ii. Neck irradiation for throat tumor, surgical section of glossopharyngeal nerve, and degenerative disease of nuclei tractus solitarius, resulting in carotid baroreceptor denervation

      c. Symptoms
         i. Severe and episodic
         ii. Hallmarks are chronic labile hypertension and tachycardia alternating with hypotension and bradycardia
         iii. Paroxysms last 3–20 minutes
         iv. Headache, diaphoresis, and tachycardia are often severe
         v. Flushing episodes may be severe but usually are associated with pallor rather than redness
         vi. Emotional lability is common, especially early, and may be associated with severe pressure elevations that respond to sedation

      d. Laboratory findings
         i. Between attacks catecholamines may be normal
         ii. During attacks plasma norepinephrine often is elevated dramatically

   iii. Mental arithmetic test reveals supranormal pressor response
   iv. Clonidine suppression test is most useful (see Appendix III)
  2. Increased intracranial pressure
  3. Posterior fossa lesions
  4. Guillain-Barré syndrome
  5. Stroke (see chapter 2, page 17)
  6. Spinal cord lesions or spinal surgery
   a. Posttraumatic spinal cord syndromes
    i. Initial spinal shock
    ii. Early orthostatic hypotension
    iii. Late autonomic dysreflexia
     (a) Delayed onset (weeks to 1 year)
     (b) Generally with complete cord lesions above T5
     (c) Attacks of severe hypertension followed by reflex bradycardia and arrhythmias
      (i) Precipitating factors
       • Gaseous or bladder distention
       • Labor in pregnancy
       • Bladder catheterization
       • Muscle spasms
      (ii) Attacks mediated by norepinephrine release in face of denervated alpha receptors, leading to severe vasoconstriction and marked systolic and diastolic hypertension
      (iii) Reflex bradycardia and arrhythmias may follow rise in pressure and be accompanied by diaphoresis and flushing above lesion
  7. Tetanus
 E. **Drugs** (Table 5)
 F. **Preeclampsia** (see Chapter 6)

TABLE 5. Drugs Reported to Cause Hypertension

Birth control pills	Venlafaxine
Licorice, carbenoxalone*	Tobacco (especially in large amounts and/or with caffeine)
Heavy metals	Cyclosporine
Monoamine oxidase inhibitors plus tyramine, sympathomimetic agents, guanadrel, buspirone, or amantadine	Chlorpromazine
Nonsteroidal anti-inflammatory drugs	Erythropoietin
Sympathomimetics (including surreptitious use and "food supplements"†)	Depo-medroxyprogesterone[16]
Tricyclic antidepressants	Conjugated estrogens/diethylstilbestrol[17]
Steroids	Topical or inhaled fluorinated steroids[18]
Excessive exogenous thyroid hormones	Cocaine, amphetamines, methylphenidate, phencyclidine
Ergotamine, dihydroergotamine, midodrine	Alcohol
Metoclopramide (with pheochromocytoma)‡	Bromocriptine (postpartum)‡
	Disulfiram with alcohol

* Licorice contains a steroid (glycyrrhetinic acid) that inhibits 11-beta hydroxysteroid dehydrogenase, leading to cortisol acting as the major endogenous mineralocorticoid because it is not metabolized to cortisone. Direct action of glycyrrhetinic acid is no longer thought to be the major cause of hypermineralocorticoidism in this syndrome.[15]

† Including ma huang (*Ephedra sinica* or Chinese ephedra), which contains ephedrine and other catecholamines.

‡ Rare causes.

G. **Acute intermittent porphyria:** may look like pheochromocytoma with

1. Abdominal pain
2. Back pain
3. Muscle weakness with normal creatine phosphokinase (CPK)
4. Postural hypotension
5. Hyponatremia
6. Fever
7. Nausea and vomiting

H. **Sleep apnea syndrome**
   1. Common in both men and women
   2. Hallmarks
      a. Daytime somnolence, especially falling asleep during activities for which alertness is important
      b. Snoring
      c. Unrestful sleep
      d. Sudden nocturnal awakening with gasping
   2. Additional features
      a. Hypertension usually persists during day
      b. Increased arrhythmias and cardiovascular mortality
      c. Some patients may have nocturnal hypotension[19]

I. **Acute hypoxemia**

III. **Approach to the Patient**[20]
   A. **History**
      1. **To detect secondary causes and exacerbating factors**
         a. Age < 35 or > 55 favors secondary hypertension
         b. Personal medical history and family history
            i. Flank trauma or flank pain may point to renal ischemia
            ii. Lack of family history may favor secondary hypertension
            iii. MEN, von Hippel-Lindau syndrome, and neurofibromatosis are associated with pheochromocytoma
         c. Medication history (also see Table 5)
            i. Including over-the-counter medications
               (a) Decongestants (e.g., nasal spray and cold remedies)
               (b) Antiasthmatic remedies (e.g., Primatene Mist)
               (c) Weight loss preparations
               (d) Nonsteroidal anti-inflammatory drugs
            ii. Herbal remedies
               (a) Herb teas used for weight loss
               (b) Other herbal preparations
         d. Personal, dietary, and social history
            i. Alcohol, particularly more than 1–2 drinks per day, may elevate arterial pressure
            ii. Smoking
               (a) Particularly when combined with caffeine and/or alcohol may exacerbate hypertension
               (b) Nicotine in tobacco may exacerbate pheochromocytoma
               (c) Most older patients with renovascular hypertension have history of smoking
            iii. Illicit drugs such as amphetamines and cocaine are important causes of hypertension
            iv. Licorice-flavored foods, tobaccos, and beverages
            v. Caffeine intake

      vi. Sodium intake

     vii. Saturated fat intake

    viii. Sexual dysfunction

     ix. Psychosocial factors

        (a) Family situation

        (b) Working conditions and employment

        (c) Level of education

  e. Review of systems

      i. Polyuria, polydipsia, or nocturia may suggest renal or endocrine disorders, especially in children; polyuria may be seen with obstructive uropathy

     ii. Weight gain, ecchymoses, edema, new acne, change in libido or behavior, or change in menstrual patterns may point to Cushing's syndrome

    iii. Oligomenorrhea and hirsutism may accompany Cushing's, thyroid, or adrenogenital syndrome

    iv. Headache, diaphoresis, palpitations, postural hypotension, flushing, and heat intolerance may suggest pheochromocytoma

2. **To assess end-organ damage**

  a. Angina or myocardial infarction (marked blood pressure reduction *may* be harmful)

  b. Transient cerebrovascular ischemic attacks (TIAs) or strokes

  c. Congestive heart failure

  d. Claudication

  e. Renal failure or history of renal disease

3. **To assess risk**

  a. Tobacco

  b. Diabetes mellitus

  c. Family history of premature death due to vascular complications

  d. Lipid disorders

  e. Age over 60 years

  f. Males or postmenopausal women

  g. History of left ventricular hypertrophy

  h. Peripheral vascular disease

  i. Weight gain

  j. Lack of physical activity

4. **To detect conditions that may benefit from specific types of treatment** (see Chapter 4)

B. **Physical examination**

1. **To detect secondary causes**

  a. General appearance

      i. Cushing's syndrome

        (a) Moon facies   (e) Purple striae

        (b) Plethora   (f) Supraclavicular fullness

        (c) Ecchymoses   (very common)

        (d) Truncal obesity   (g) Hirsutism

     ii. Coarctation of aorta

        (a) Leg pressure < 10 mm higher than arm pressure

        (b) 10-mm differential between arms

      (c) Unequal arm development or reduced development of lower extremities uncommon but much more specific than blood pressure inequality

      (d) Grade 2–3/6 systolic murmur best heard over posterior left interscapular area (common)

      (e) Systolic or continuous murmurs, which may be heard on either side anteriorly, are less common

   iii. Marfanoid habitus in MEN type III (type IIb)

   iv. Hirsutism with or without genital virilism or infantilism may be clue to adrenogenital syndrome

   v. Pallor of extremities (pheochromocytoma)

b. **Blood pressure**

   i. Taken in both upper extremities, supine, and after standing at least 2 minutes and in leg if < 35 years old

   ii. In essential hypertension, diastolic pressure rises on standing; decrease suggests secondary hypertension

   iii. Unequal blood pressure in arms or leg pressure ≤ arm pressure—more commonly due to atherosclerosis than coarctation

   iv. Osler's maneuver

      (a) Palpable brachial or radial artery with blood pressure cuff inflated above systolic to detect pseudohypertension

      (b) Sensitivity of test controversial[21]

   v. Isolated systolic hypertension may be due to

      (a) Severe anemia　　　(d) Paget's disease of bone

      (b) Hyperthyroidism　　(e) Arteriosclerosis

      (c) Aortic insufficiency

c. **Fundi:** retinal hemangiomas in von Hippel-Lindau syndrome

d. **Carotid bruits** suggest that atherosclerotic renal artery stenosis may be more likely

e. **Extracardiac bruits**

   i. In chest may suggest coarctation

   ii. In abdomen may suggest renal artery stenosis

      (a) Best heard just lateral to midline above umbilicus or in flanks

      (b) Systolic alone is not specific

      (c) Diastolic components more specific

      (d) Bruits occur in 40% of patients with atherosclerotic renal artery stenosis

   iii. Cerebellar hemangioblastoma in von Hippel-Lindau syndrome

f. **Palpation of abdomen**

   i. Polycystic kidney disease

   ii. Renal cysts of von Hippel-Lindau syndrome

   iii. Rarely vigorous palpation may cause pheochromocytoma paroxysm

g. **Café-au-lait spots**

   i. Localized flat areas of hyperpigmentation 0.5–12 cm in diameter

   ii. More than 5 spots over 1.5 cm (0.5 cm in children) in diameter suggest possible neurofibromatosis and associated pheochromocytoma or fibromuscular dysplasia

2. **To assess end-organs:** hypertension-related changes reflect increased risk from hypertension

a. Fundi
b. Cardiac status
c. Neurologic status

d. Pulses, check for aneurysms
e. Edema, rales, jugular venous pressure

3. **Examination relevant to systolic hypertension**
   a. Thyroid
   b. Tremor

   c. Pallor
   d. Aortic insufficiency
4. **Technique of blood pressure determination:** if initial office readings elevated, repeat after several minutes
   a. Continue this procedure every 5 minutes until consecutive pressures are similar
   b. This technique improves diagnostic accuracy and reduces false-positive elevations ("white-coat" hypertension)[22]

C. **Basic initial laboratory evaluation**
   1. **Chemistry panel**
      a. Hypercalcemia
         i. Hyperparathyroidism
         ii. MEN
         iii. Pheochromocytoma
      b. Hyperglycemia
         i. Cushing's syndrome
         ii. Pheochromocytoma
         iii. Acromegaly
         iv. Coexistent primary diabetes mellitus
      c. Electrolyte abnormalities (see E.5. below)
   2. Urinalysis
   3. Electrocardiogram
   4. Chest radiograph
   5. Hematocrit
   6. **Absolute minimal evaluation** should include
      a. Urine dipstick
      b. Hematocrit
      c. Potassium

      d. Creatinine
      e. Electrocardiogram

D. **Additional laboratory tests**
   1. Echocardiogram
      a. Not routinely needed
      b. May be useful in making decision to treat
   2. Home blood pressure monitoring
      a. Self-taken: especially useful in patients with negative family history and labile hypertension and those with apparent medication intolerance
      b. Ambulatory monitoring
         i. Useful in select cases
            (a) Nocturnal syncope with no Holter monitor abnormalities[23]
            (b) If patient-reported home readings do not explain findings or "white-coat" hypertension is suspected
            (c) Confirmation of nocturnal blood pressure control
            (d) Assessment of symptoms thought to be pressure-related but not revealed by home readings
            (e) Unexplained end-organ damage (e.g., left ventricular hypertrophy)

      (f) Autonomic dysfunction

      (g) Drug resistance or hypotension on antihypertensive drugs

    ii. Normal values

      (a) ≤ 118/72 for 24-hour average

      (b) ≤ 123/76 daytime average

    iii. Ambulatory hypertension

      (a) 134/87 24-hour average

      (b) 140/90 daytime average has been cited as abnormal[24]

      (c) 130/85 mean daytime average has been found in recent study to correlate with mean clinic blood pressure of 140/90 and therefore may be used to define hypertension more accurately[25]

  3. Renal ultrasound in patients with symptoms of obstruction (including urinary frequency or polyuria), patients with elevated serum creatinines, and all hypertensive children

E. **Secondary hypertension: work-up and triggers for further evaluation**

  1. **Onset at age < 25 or > 50** suggests work-up for secondary hypertension, particularly

    a. Renal parenchymal disease

    b. Renovascular hypertension

  2. **Abdominal bruit**

    a. Work-up for renal artery stenosis (see Appendix IV) if continuous (both systolic and diastolic components)

    b. Isolated systolic bruit is not sufficient evidence by itself to mandate work-up for renovascular hypertension, particularly in older people

  3. **Resistant** (more difficult-to-control) hypertension without clear explanation: appropriate possibilities based on history and physical examination (Table 6)

TABLE 6.   Causes of Labile and Resistant Hypertension

1. Dietary noncompliance	20. Rapid drug inactivation (e.g., hydralazine + smoking or rifampin + propranolol)
2. Drug noncompliance	21. Vasculitis or Raynaud's phenomenon
3. Primary labile hypertension	22. Inappropriate combinations (e.g., methyldopa + beta blocker)
4. Hyperthyroidism	
5. Urinary retention or obstruction (even unilateral)[26]	23. Strokes or cord lesions
6. Transient ischemic attacks	24. Alcohol or alcohol withdrawal
7. Postural drop in blood pressure	25. Malignant hypertension
8. Renal artery stenosis	26. Fluid retention reset syndrome (initially effective regimen fails in patient on adrenal inhibitor, vasodilator, or both, leading to compensatory volume expansion)
9. Combined tobacco and caffeine (particularly in high doses)	
10. Drug-related causes (Table 7)	
11. Pseudohypertension	27. Hyperaldosteronism
12. Cardiac causes	28. Scleroderma
13. Office or "white-coat" hypertension	29. Angina pectoris
14. Sleep apnea	30. Wrong cuff size
15. Pheochromocytoma	31. Myocardial infarction
16. Renal failure (volume- or renin-dependent)	32. Acute intermittent porphyria
17. Acute hypoxemia	33. Aortic valve replacement
18. Hyperinsulinemia or insulin resistance	34. Coarctation of aorta
	35. Coronary bypass (pressor reflex)[27,28]
19. Severe (especially chronic) pain	36. Carcinoid syndrome
	37. Acromegaly

TABLE 7. Drug-related Causes of Labile and Resistant Hypertension

1. Nonsteroidal anti-inflammatory drugs antagonize all antihypertensives except perhaps central alpha blockers and calcium channel blockers
2. Birth control pills
3. Steroids
4. Tricyclic antidepressants, especially with methyldopa or clonidine
5. Sympathomimetics, especially decongestants with beta blockers
6. Failure to use diuretic, especially with volume-expanding antihypertensive medications or even mild azotemia
7. Inadequate dosage or inadequate frequency (e.g., once-daily ACE inhibitor [breakthrough hypertension[29]])
8. Use of beta blocker in patient withdrawn from clonidine[30]
9. Cyclosporine
10. Erythropoietin
11. Excessive doses of thyroid hormone
12. Sympathomimetic illicit drugs (cocaine, amphetamines, phencyclidine)
13. Drug interactions (see Appendix VIII)
14. Chronic narcotic use, especially in variable doses and schedules for chronic pain

4. **Postural hypotension**
    a. Pheochromocytoma
    b. Porphyria
    c. Renal artery stenosis
5. **Stigmata or classic history** leads to appropriate work-up
    a. Moon facies, plethora, hyperglycemia, supraclavicular fullness, purple striae, edema, buffalo hump, truncal obesity: **Cushing's syndrome** (see Appendix I)
    b. **Hypokalemia without other stigmata**
        i. Hallmark of primary hyperaldosteronism (see Appendix II). Additional clues to hyperaldosteronism include
            (a) Mild hypernatremia
            (b) Mild metabolic acidosis
            (c) Hypomagnesemia
            (d) Lack of edema
        ii. Common in renovascular hypertension
        iii. Seen also in
            (a) Malignant hypertension
            (b) Cushing's syndrome
            (c) Liddle syndrome
                (i) Simulates hypermineralocorticoidism with hypokalemic alkalosis and hypertension
                (ii) Defect in sodium-potassium exchange mechanism in renal tubule
                (iii) Accompanied by suppression of both renin and aldosterone without presence of abnormal steroid
        iv. Although adrenal hyperplasia may occur without hypokalemia, adenomas usually do not
        v. Hypokalemia of mild severity (≥ 3.0)
            (a) Not unusual in patients on diuretic therapy. Therefore, in **patients taking diuretics** mildly depressed serum potassium alone is not sufficient grounds to justify further evaluation

      (b) Hypokalemia in patients taking diuretics frequently due to excessive salt intake or excessive diuretic usage

      (c) In **absence of diuretic therapy** or another obvious cause, **even mild hypokalemia** should lead to consideration of secondary hypertension

  c. Palpitations, headaches, anxiety attacks, unusual sweating, hyperglycemia, weight loss; familial MEN, or multiple café-au-lait spots: suspect **pheochromocytoma**

  d. Coarse facies, diaphoresis, acral enlargement, hypertrichosis, voice change, paresthesias, glucose intolerance, goiter, fibromata (many features similar to minoxidil side effects): **acromegaly**

  e. Episodic hypertension, back or abdominal pain, constipation, muscle weakness with normal CPK (paroxysms of hypertension last longer than in pheochromocytoma); fever, leukocytosis, postural hypotension, nausea, vomiting, sinus tachycardia, syndrome of inappropriate antidiuretic hormone secretion, neuropathy: **acute intermittent porphyria**

  f. Consider **renal artery stenosis** work-up (see Appendix IV) with

    i. Age < 25 or > 50
    ii. Young women (fibromuscular dysplasia)
    iii. Severe hypertension
    iv. Malignant hypertension
    v. Continuous bruit
    vi. Orthostatic drop in diastolic pressure
    vii. Absence of family history of essential hypertension
    viii. Neurofibromatosis

  g. **Urinary obstruction or retention** should be excluded in patients with

    i. Hyperkalemia
    ii. Polyuria
    iii. Frequency
    iv. Nocturia
    v. Diabetes mellitus
    vi. Spinal or neuromuscular disorders

6. Evaluation of patients suspected of having **renovascular hypertension**

  a. To determine whether surgical correction is indicated in hypertensive patients without azotemia, renal vein renin is no longer recommended because newer studies indicate that it not sufficiently accurate[31]

  b. Clinical judgment now used for deciding appropriateness of correction

  c. Correction is indicated in azotemic patients with renal artery stenosis to preserve renal function, regardless of whether they have renal artery stenosis-mediated hypertension

  d. **Screening tests**

    i. **Captopril renography** or gadolinium-enhanced magnetic resonance angiography (GEMRA) (preferred initial screening test) (Table 8 and Appendix IV)

TABLE 8. Captopril Renography[33,34]

1. Continue all usual medications except ACE inhibitors, which should be stopped 24 hr before test
2. Give 3 glasses of water at home
3. Give 50 mg of crushed captopril by mouth
4. Do DTPA renography 1 hour later while replacing urinary losses
5. Positive tests are *either*   • Peak activity ≥ 11 minutes *or*   • GFR ratio > 1.5

DTPA = [99m]diethylenetriaminepentaacetate; GFR = glomerular filtration rate.

TABLE 9. Captopril Test Protocol*

1. Measure plasma renin activity and blood pressure with patient sitting
2. Administer 50 mg of crushed captopril by mouth
3. Check plasma renin activity 1 hour later
4. Criteria for positive test (**all** must be satisfied)
   - Stimulated renin of 10–12 µg/L/hr
   - Increase in renin by 10 µg/L/hr
   - Increase in renin by 150% or 400% if baseline < 3 µg/L/hr

* Avoid sodium restriction before test.

    ii. **Captopril test** (Table 9)
       (a) Of limited utility by itself
       (b) More useful with isotope renography but still not completely reliable
       (c) Not recommended as sole screening procedure
       (d) Accuracy may be improved with sodium repletion and prior discontinuation of medications affecting renin-angiotensin system directly (beta blockers, ACE inhibitors, diuretics)[32]
    iii. **Direct arteriography (with digital subtraction if possible):** favored over screening tests in cases with high clinical suspicion without contraindications to procedure and when either stent placement or surgery will be performed (see Appendix IV)
    iv. **Magnetic resonance angiography**
       (a) Good for main vessels
       (b) Not as good for non-main arteries
       (c) GEMRA preferred

REFERENCES

1. Preston R, Singer I, Epstein M: Renal parenchymal hypertension: Current concepts of pathogenesis and management. Arch Intern Med 1996;156:602–611.
2. National High Blood Pressure Working Group: 1995 Update of the working group reports on chronic renal failure and renovascular hypertension. Arch Intern Med 1996;156: 1938–1947.
3. Svetkey LP, Saadon K, et al: Similar prevalence of renovascular hypertension in selected blacks and whites. Hypertension 1991;17:678–683.
4. Rich GM, Ullick S, Cook S, et al: Glucocorticoid-remediable aldosteronism in a large kindred: Clinical spectrum and diagnosis using a characteristic biochemical phenotype. Ann Intern Med 1992;116:813–820.
5. Gordon RD: Syndrome of hypertension and hyperkalemia with normal glomerular filtration rate. Hypertension 1986;8:93.
6. Wang C, Chan TK, Yeung RT, et al: The effect of triamterene and sodium intake on renin, aldosterone, and erythrocyte sodium transport in Liddle's syndrome. J Clin Endocrinol Metab 1981;52:1027–1032.
7. Mutoh S, Hirayam H, Ueda S, et al: Pseudohyperaldosteronism (Liddle's syndrome): A case report. J Urol 1986;135:557–558.
8. Nakada T, Koike H, Akiya T, et al: Liddle's syndrome, uncommon form of hyporeninemic hypoaldosteronism: Functional and histopathological studies. J Urol 1987;137:636–640.
9. Takeuchi K, Abe K, Sato M, et al: Plasma aldosterone level in a female case of pseudohypoaldosteronism (Liddle's syndrome). Endocr J 1989;36:167–173.
10. Fine RN: Clinical quiz. Pediatr Nephrol 1990;4:705–706.
11. Stewart PM, Corrie JET, Shackleton CHL, Edwards CRW: Syndrome of apparent mineralocorticoid excess: A defect in the cortisol-cortisone shuttle. J Clin Invest 1988;82:340–349.
12. Ulick S, Tedde R, Mantem F: Pathogenesis of the type 2 variant of the syndrome of apparent mineralocorticoid excess. J Clin Endocrinol Metab 1990;70:49–54.

13. Ulick S, Tedde R, Wang JZ: Defective ring A reduction of cortisol as the major metabolic error in the syndrome of apparent mineralocorticoid excess. J Clin Endocrinol Metab 1992;74:593–599.

14. Yi J, Bakris GL: Pheochromocytoma. In Current Diagnosis 9. Philadelphia, W.B. Saunders, 1997, pp 794–798.

15. Farese RV, Biglieri EG, Shackleton CHL, et al: Licorice induced hypermineralocorticoidism. N Engl J Med 1991;325:1223–1227.

16. Leiman G: Depo-medroxyprogesterone as a contraceptive agent: Its effect on weight and blood pressure. Am J Obstet Gynecol 1972;114:97–102.

17. Crane MG, Harris JB: Estrogens and hypertension: Effect of discontinuing estrogens on blood pressure, exchangeable sodium and the renin-aldosterone system. Am J Med Sci 1978;276:33–55.

18. Vasconey F, Erez-Garcia R, et al: Hypermineralocorticoidism syndrome secondary to topical application of 9-alpha floroprednisolone. Med Clin (Barcelona) 1980;75:430.

19. McGinty D, Beahm E, Stern N, et al: Nocturnal hypotension in older men with sleep-related breathing disorders. Chest 1988;94:305–311.

20. Slataper RM, Bakris GL: Secondary hypertension. In Taylor R (ed): Difficult Diagnosis II. Philadelphia, W.B. Saunders, 1992, pp 403–411.

21. Setaro JF, Black HR: Refractory hypertension. N Engl J Med 1993;27:543–547.

22. Fagard RH, Staessen JA, Thijs L: Prediction of cardiac structure and function by repeated clinic and ambulatory blood pressure. Hypertension 1997;29(1 Pt 1):22–29.

23. Grin JM, McCaber EJ, White WB: Management of hypertension after ambulatory blood pressure monitoring. Ann Intern Med 1993;118:833–837.

24. Staessen JA, Fagard RH, Linjen PJ, et al: Mean and range of the ambulatory blood pressure in normotensive subjects from a meta-analysis of 23 studies. Am J Cardiol 1991;67:723.

25. Mancia G, Sega R, Bravi C, et al: Ambulatory blood pressure normality: Results from the PAMELA study. J Hypertens 1995;13:1377–1390.

26. Weidmann P, Beretta-Piccoli C, Hirsh D, et al: Curable hypertension associated with unilateral hydronephrosis. Studies on the role of circulating renin. Ann Intern Med 1977;87:437–440.

27. Dustin HP, Tarazi RC: Cardiogenic hypertension. Annu Rev Med 1978;29:485–493.

28. Estafanous FG, Tarazi RC: Systemic arterial hypertension associated with cardiac surgery. Am J Cardiol 1980;46:685–694.

29. Neutel JM, Smith DHG: Breakthrough hypertension. Cardiovasc Res Rep 1991;12:38–40.

30. Bailey RR, Neale TJ: Rapid clonidine withdrawal and blood pressure overshoot exaggerated by beta-blockade. BMJ 1976;1:942–943.

31. Rudnick MR, Maxwell MH: Limitations of renin assays. In Narins RG (ed): Controversies in Nephrology and Hypertension. New York, Churchill Livingstone, 1984, pp 123–160.

32. McCarthy JE, Weder AB: The captopril test and renovascular hypertension: A cautionary tale. Arch Intern Med 1990;150:493–495.

33. Setaro JF, Saddler MC, Chen CC, et al: Simplified captopril renography in diagnosis and treatment of renal artery stenosis. Hypertension 1991;18:289–298.

34. Davidson R, Wilcox CS: Diagnostic usefulness of renal scanning after angiotensin converting enzyme inhibitors [editorial]. Hypertension 1991;18:299–303.

CHAPTER 4

Treatment of the Hypertensive Patient

I. **When to Treat**

   A. Anyone with **systolic pressure ≥ 140 mmHg and/or diastolic pressure ≥ 90 mmHg without contraindication** such as acute stroke[1] (see page 17) or postural hypotension should be treated

   B. JNC VI recommendations suggest individualizing goals based on coexisting conditions and additional risk factors (see Chapter 2, Tables 3 and 4)

   C. Benefit in reduction of morbidity and mortality with mild hypertension is small but significant[2]

   D. **Treatment of isolated systolic hypertension** (ISH) in elderly is beneficial[2]

      1. Treatment more important with additional risk factors

      2. Recent recommendation is to treat patients whose systolic pressure consistently averages 140 mmHg or more[3]

      3. Use drugs with lowest risk of serious adverse reactions

         a. Avoid methyldopa, beta blockers, reserpine, ganglionic blockers, nifedipine

         b. Consider low-dose thiazides[2] (preferred), long-acting calcium channel blockers (recommended by JNC VI), or ACE inhibitors[3]

      4. Pseudohypertension must be excluded

      5. Orthostatic changes of dramatic degree preclude initiation of therapy and should be watched for carefully during therapy[4]

      6. ISH with low diastolic pressure is associated with even higher cardiovascular risk; lower systolic pressure lowers risk even if diastolic pressure drops even further

   E. **Ambulatory blood pressure monitoring**

      1. Potential usefulness[5]

         a. Distinguishing "white-coat" hypertension from sustained disease

         b. Confirming 24-hour control

         c. Studying significance of labile hypertension

         d. Studying nocturnal blood pressure

         e. Drug-resistant hypertension

         f. Hypotensive symptoms without apparent explanation

      2. Better correlation with end-organ damage than casual office readings as of the time of this writing

      3. Concerns that such technology will be overutilized have not been supported by data[6]

      4. Established norms: mean of < 135/85 mmHg in daytime hours, but norm varies with age[7]

   F. **Pressure goal**

      1. **Generally 120–130/75–85 mmHg**

      2. In certain populations lower pressure goals have shown benefit

         a. In patients with azotemia lower pressures were associated with slower progression of renal disease, if proteinuria was present[6,8,9]

         b. In patients with congestive heart failure[10]

         c. For prevention of stroke[11]

         d. Diabetes mellitus (see pages 57–58)

      3. Concerns about dropping pressure too low

         a. J curve has **not** been seen in clinical trials with goals of systolic hypertension < 140 mmHg or diastolic hypertension < 90 mmHg. This finding recently was supported by the HOT study of over 19,000 patients and the UKPDS trial.[12]

      b. Mortality associated with lower pressures, when seen, occurred in placebo arms of trials as well as treatment arms; thus, therapy is less likely to be culprit

      c. If relevant to any population, it is most likely in patients with both preexisting coronary artery disease and hypertension

      d. Current goals in ISH[5]

        i. About 140 mmHg if blood pressure initially > 160 mmHg

        ii. 20 mmHg lower than initially if initial pressure < 160 mmHg

II. Nondrug Therapy

A. Attempt in all patients

B. Stress reduction

1. Avoid unnecessary stress
2. Rare cases require job change
3. No evidence of long-term benefit of biofeedback

C. Diet

1. Moderate salt restriction = 2 gm sodium (5 gm NaCl)

    a. At least 50% of patients respond to salt restriction without drugs (at least partially; average reduction = 4 mmHg)

    b. Even in nonresponders it often markedly potentiates effect of medications

    c. Assess compliance with 24-hr urine sodium (valid even in patients taking diuretics, if they were started at least 3 weeks previously)

    d. Greatest effect in older patients, African-Americans, and patients with more severe hypertension

    e. Important in patients with diabetes, in whom high-salt diet may partly reverse benefits of ACE inhibitors or calcium channel blockers on progression of proteinuria[13,14] and in whom sodium retention may be factor in pathogenesis of hyperfiltration and hypertension[15]

    f. Also of greater importance in patients with renal parenchymal disease[16]

2. Higher calcium diet

    a. Controversial

    b. Most justifiable in patients at risk for osteoporosis

    c. May worsen calcium kidney stone disease

3. Attainment of ideal body weight lowers blood pressure even without salt restriction

4. Low-cholesterol, low-saturated fat diet reduces other risk factors but has little effect on blood pressure

5. Isotonic exercise within reason

6. Decreased ethanol intake: < 3 drinks/day (optimal)

7. High potassium diet (sufficient to maintain normal serum K; intake should be ≥ 60 mEq/day[17,18])

    a. Included in JNC VI recommendations[5]

    b. Should **not** be recommended to any patient who is

      i. Hyperkalemic before therapy

      ii. Taking ACE inhibitors, potassium-sparing diuretics, or beta blockers if significant renal insufficiency is present (i.e., creatinine clearance < 35 cc/min or serum creatinine > 3; use caution even with lesser degrees of renal impairment if patient is taking more than one of these three classes of drugs)

    c. May lower pressure further in patients taking antihypertensives[19]

8. Increasing celery intake (6–8 stalks/day) *may* reduce elevated arterial pressure[20,21]

9. "Dash" diet, which incorporates high potassium, high magnesium, and high calcium with low sodium, may reduce systolic blood pressure by 10 mmHg or more[5]

C. Eliminate hypertension-worsening drugs (see Table 5, page 29)

1. Nonsteroidal anti-inflammatory drugs (NSAIDs)
2. Steroids
3. Birth control pills
4. Sympathomimetics
5. Reduce tobacco use (reduces risks of coronary disease, stroke, subarachnoid hemorrhage, malignant hypertension, cancer, sudden death, and emphysema)

III. **Drug Therapy** (see also Appendix V)

A. **Diuretics**

1. **Thiazides and thiazide-like agents**

a. Examples
   i. Thiazides (e.g., hydrochlorothiazide, chlorthalidone)
   ii. Indolines (e.g., indapamide)
   iii. Quinazolines (e.g., metolazone)

b. Generally effective and well tolerated—many patients cannot be adequately controlled without diuretic; avoiding these agents in such patients is clearly harmful

c. Drugs of choice for patients with recurrent **kidney stones** caused by hypercalciuria

d. **Dosage**
   i. Should be initiated in small doses (e.g., 12.5 mg hydrochlorothiazide/day, preferred)
   ii. Maximal dose: 25 mg hydrochlorothiazide/day for control of hypertension
   iii. At lower doses, potassium levels below 3 are more likely to result from noncompliance with salt restriction or from secondary hypertension (see Potassium balance below)
   iv. Higher doses more likely to be associated with adverse effects and do **not** lower blood pressure further in most patients
   v. Higher doses are often needed for treatment of hypercalciuria
   vi. Higher doses associated with
      (a) Hypokalemia   (d) Hyperuricemia
      (b) Hyperlipidemia   (e) Insulin resistance
      (c) Hypomagnesemia

e. **Potassium balance**
   i. As rule, potassium is not affected in a clinically important way by small doses of currently recommended diuretics (unless patient ingests high-salt diet, which potentiates kaliuresis). **Note:** best blood pressure control is found when serum potassium levels are normalized (≥ 4.0)
   ii. Slight reduction of serum potassium need not be treated except[22–26]
      (a) When patient is symptomatic
      (b) When patient is taking digitalis

      (c) With history of arrhythmias

      (d) With history of ischemic heart disease

      (e) With abnormal electrocardiogram

      (f) Prior to anesthesia

      (g) With liver disease

      (h) With carbohydrate intolerance (?)

    iii. When hypokalemia occurs in patients taking diuretics, it usually does so within first 2 weeks of therapy (assuming constant sodium intake); new-onset hypokalemia after that time suggests

      (a) Increase in dietary sodium intake and/or

      (b) Change in diuretic dose and/or

      (c) Unrelated cause of hypokalemia

    iv. Significant hypokalemia while patient is taking diuretics may be clue to

      (a) Noncompliance with sodium restriction

      (b) Inadequate nutrition

      (c) Renal artery stenosis

      (d) Hypermineralocorticoidism

  f. **Hyperlipidemia and diuretics**

    i. No evidence indicates that long-term hyperlipidemia of any significance results from currently recommended doses of diuretics

    ii. Indapamide does not seem to cause changes in serum lipids

2. **Loop diuretics**

  a. Examples

    i. Furosemide   iii. Ethacrynic acid

    ii. Bumetanide   iv. Torsemide

  b. Short duration of action mandates more frequent administration

  c. Many adverse effects more common than with thiazides

  d. Almost always required with

    i. Congestive heart failure

    ii. Renal insufficiency, especially with concomitant vasodilator therapy

3. **Potassium-sparing diuretics**

  a. Increased risk of hyperkalemia, especially

    i. Without other diuretics

    ii. With coadministration of ACE inhibitors

    iii. With coadministration of beta blockers

    iv. With NSAIDs

    v. With potassium administration

    vi. With diabetes mellitus

    vii. With renal diseases

  b. Available drugs

    i. Spironolactone

      (a) Drug of choice in hyperaldosteronism

      (b) Can be used to prevent potassium loss

    ii. Triamterene

      (a) Also used to prevent hypokalemia

      (b) No intrinsic antihypertensive activity

      (c) Occasionally forms triamterene kidney stones

     iii. Amiloride
- (a) May have theoretical advantage over other potassium-sparing diuretics in diabetic patients[27]
- (b) Although usual maximal dose is 10 mg/day, doses up to 40 mg/day are often required for treating primary aldosteronism, and high doses of amiloride are usually better tolerated than high doses of spironolactone

B. **Adrenergic antagonists**
1. **Agents active at alpha receptors**
   a. **Central alpha-2 agonists:** inhibit central nervous system outflow to preganglionic sympathetic fibers
      i. Clonidine
         - (a) Usually best given twice daily
         - (b) No orthostasis because, although resting heart rate may fall, baroreceptor reflex is preserved
         - (c) Reduce initial dose in elderly patients and in patients with renal insufficiency, starting with 0.1 mg **once daily**
         - (d) Severe rebound hypertension may occur if drug stopped suddenly
      ii. Methyldopa
         - (a) Twice-daily dosing usually adequate
         - (b) Orthostasis may occur, because of effect on primary vasomotor fibers, which control arteriolar tone (therefore, baroreceptor arc is impaired)
      iii. Guanabenz: may produce milder side effects than clonidine
      iv. Guanfacine: similar to guanabenz
   b. **Selective alpha-1 blockers**
      i. Block norepinephrine action at affected cell receptors
      ii. Potential for first-dose orthostasis
      iii. Drugs of choice in patients with urinary retention due to prostatism
      iv. Agents
         - (a) Prazosin: relatively weak drug that requires dosing 2 or 3 times/day
         - (b) Terazosin: twice-daily dose required for blood pressure control
         - (c) Doxazosin: only one daily dose required
   c. **Nonselective alpha blockers**
      i. Generally avoided in uncomplicated essential hypertension because of side effects and tolerance
      ii. Both presynaptic and postsynaptic receptors are blocked, with accumulation of norepinephrine at synapse (which normally gives feedback to stop further adrenergic output). Increasing norepinephrine release leads to escape from antihypertensive action of drug
      iii. Useful in
         - (a) Pheochromocytoma
         - (b) Rebound hypertension
         - (c) Monoamine oxidase inhibitor crisis
2. **Postganglionic nerve ending-acting agents**
   a. Guanethidine and guanadrel
      i. Block norepinephrine release at nerve ending

ii. Have greater effect on systolic pressure

iii. Because of orthostasis and gastrointestinal side effects, rarely used in U.S. today

b. Reserpine

i. Prevents norepinephrine storage

ii. Causes most side effects of guanethidine *plus* depression but less orthostasis and greater diastolic control

iii. Other newer, equally effective, and better tolerated drugs are now widely available

3. **Beta blockers** (see Appendix V)

a. **Common to all beta blockers**

i. Sudden withdrawal may result in rebound hypertension, angina, or myocardial infarction, even in patients with no history of coronary disease

ii. Particularly useful for reversing secondary effects of other antihypertensives that limit their effectiveness, such as

(a) Diuretics (which cause renin to increase)

(b) Direct vasodilators (which cause tachycardia)

iii. None of these drugs is safe for asthmatics with significant bronchospasm

b. **Nonselective beta blockers:** include propranolol, timolol, and nadolol

c. **Nonselective beta blockers with intrinsic sympathomimetic activity (ISA)**

i. Include pindolol and penbutol

ii. Preferred for patients with symptomatic bradycardia

iii. Do not affect serum lipids

iv. Unlike other beta blockers, may not be cardioprotective after myocardial infarction

d. **Selective beta-1 blockers without ISA**

i. Include atenolol, metoprolol, and betaxolol

ii. May be slightly less likely to precipitate bronchospasm

iii. In practice, selectivity is not complete and should not be depended on in severe asthmatics

iv. Better choice in patients with chronic pulmonary obstructive disease **who require beta blocker**, provided that they have history of mild or no bronchospasm

v. Also may be appropriate in diabetics who will benefit from their effects (e.g., after myocardial infarction)

(a) Less likely to exacerbate hypertension during hypoglycemia and may not mask all symptoms of condition **provided that they are given in low doses**

(b) Lose selectivity at higher doses

e. **Selective beta-1 blockers with ISA**

i. Main example: acebutolol

ii. Like nonselective agents with ISA, may not be cardioprotective after myocardial infarction

C. **Direct vasodilators**

1. **Hydralazine**

a. Potent arterial vasodilator

    b. No action on venous capacitance vessels

    c. No postural changes (due to lack of action on venous capacitance vessels)

    d. Compensatory tachycardia generally requires simultaneous use of beta blockers or central alpha-2 agonists

    e. Limiting dose to 300 mg/day minimizes chance of developing lupus-like syndrome

2. **Minoxidil**

    a. One of most potent antihypertensives

    b. Requires simultaneous use of **loop diuretic and beta blocker or central alpha agonist**

    c. Generally reserved for patients presenting with **accelerated or malignant hypertension**

    d. Great utility in **resistant hypertension**

    e. Virtually any hypertensive patient can be controlled with this drug when used in combination with diuretic and adrenergic antagonist

    f. Hirsutism in most patients; females require use of depilatory

    g. Uncommon but serious risks of hemorrhagic pericarditis and tamponade

    h. Rare cases of progressive pulmonary fibrosis

D. **ACE inhibitors** (Table 10)

1. **Examples**

    a. Benazepril (Lotensin)

    b. Captopril (Capoten and others)

    c. Enalapril (Vasotec)

    d. Fosinopril (Monopril)

    e. Lisinopril (Zestril, Prinivil)

    f. Moexipril (Univasc)

    g. Ramipril (Altace)

    h. Trandolapril (Mavik)

    i. Quinapril (Accupril)

2. Lower side-effect profile compared with most other antihypertensive drugs, except perhaps angiotensin receptor blockers

3. **Most common side effects and adverse reactions**

    a. Profound hypotension when renin is activated

      i. Severe congestive heart failure

      ii. Prior diuretic therapy

      iii. Volume depletion or severe salt restriction

    b. Azotemia when renal perfusion is renin-dependent

      i. Solitary kidney with renal artery stenosis

      ii. Renal artery stenosis in kidney transplant

      iii. Bilateral renal artery stenosis

      iv. Some hypertensive azotemic patients without renal artery stenosis[28]

    c. Life-threatening hyperkalemia: the more coexisting factors, the more likely the patient will become hyperkalemic

      i. Potassium supplements

      ii. Diabetes mellitus

      iii. Urinary obstruction

      iv. Interstitial nephritis

      v. Beta blockers

      vi. Potassium-sparing diuretics

      vii. NSAIDs

    d. Intractable cough may occur with any ACE inhibitor

      i. 20% incidence in the general population

      ii. Most common in patients with DD ACE genotype

TABLE 10. Differences Between ACE Inhibitors Based on Pharmacology and Clinical Trial Evidence (Bullets are Favorable Characteristics of the Particular Category Additive to Those in Previous Category)

Benazepril Lisinopril Captopril Perindopril Cilazapril Quinapril Enalapril Ramipril Fosinopril Trandolapril	Benazepril Lisinopril Captopril Ramipril Enalapril Trandolapril	Ramipril Trandolapril
ACE inhibitor Lowers blood pressure Lowers proteinuria	Ace inhibitor Lowers blood pressure Lowers proteinuria *plus* • Reduces mortality in CHF • Reduces nephropathy progression	Ace inhibitor Lowers blood pressure Lowers proteinuria Reduces mortality in CHF Reduces nephropathy progression *plus* • Tissue selectivity • Bioavailability > 50% • Once-daily dosing • Dual mode of excretion

4. **Serious adverse effects (much less frequent)**
   a. Severe angioedema is probably most common (incidence < 1%); more common in women and African-Americans
   b. Agranulocytosis may occur with any ACE inhibitor (rarely), especially in patients with collagen vascular disease
   c. Severe dermatologic complications (rare)
   d. Membranous nephropathy with nephrotic syndromes at **very high doses** (e.g., > 500 mg/day of captopril); not reported at currently used doses
5. Effects in patients with diabetes mellitus
   a. Attenuate rise in microalbuminuria[29–32]
   b. Delay time to end-stage renal disease[17–20]
   c. Extra caution required in diabetics
      i. If proteinuria worsens, consider
         (a) Noncompliance with salt restriction
         (b) Other renal diseases: up to 30% of type II diabetics with worsening proteinuria have other glomerular diseases, such as focal glomerulosclerosis or IgA nephropathy
      ii. Hyperkalemia is commonly precipitated
      iii. Microalbuminuria or gross proteinuria should be quantified before and during use of ACE inhibitors
6. Differ in spectrum of clinical characteristics (see Table 10)
E. **Angiotensin II receptor blockers**
   1. **Examples:** losartan, valsartan, irbesartan, candesartan, and telmisartan
   2. **Common adverse effects**
      a. Expect somewhat fewer adverse effects than from ACE inhibitors in patients with azotemia, renal artery stenosis, congestive heart failure
         i. Currently recommended as alternative therapy to ACE inhibitors for congestive heart failure by JNC VI and supported by recent study comparing losartan to captopril[33]

   ii. Data from two ongoing trials in diabetic nephropathy not available at the time of this writing

  b. Fewest nonrenal side effects of any antihypertensive drug class

   i. Hyperkalemia less frequent than with ACE inhibitors but **may raise serum potassium levels**

    (a) Most common in patients with renal insufficiency and declining renal function

    (b) More likely when other drugs that potentiate hyperkalemia are given simultaneously (e.g., potassium-sparing diuretics or beta blockers)

   ii. Nasal congestion occurs in some patients

   iii. Rare serious allergic reactions and angioedema-like reactions similar to those with ACE inhibitors have been reported

   iv. Cough does not occur more often than with placebo (unlike ACE inhibitors)

F. **Calcium channel antagonists** (Table 11)

 1. **Examples**

  a. **Nondihydropyridine calcium blockers** (nonDHP CCBs)

   i. Verapamil

    (a) Most negatively inotropic

    (b) Most constipating

    (c) Least likely to cause orthostatic hypotension

    (d) Least likely to cause peripheral edema

   ii. Diltiazem: intermediate in effects between dihydropyridine blockers and verapamil

  b. **Dihydropyridine calcium blockers** (DHP CCBs)

   i. Nifedipine

    (a) Most severe orthostasis

    (b) Most severe edema

    (c) Most severe tachycardia

    (d) Most potent dihydropyridine

   ii. Amlodipine

   iii. Felodipine

   iv. Isradipine

   v. Nisoldipine

   vi. Lacidipine

   vii. Manidipine

   viii. Nitrendipine

 2. **Characteristics**

  a. Major advantage: lack of serious side effects in vast majority of patients

  b. Usage limited by constipation, especially in elderly (particularly with verapamil)

  c. Annoying edema due to local effects occurs predominantly with dihydropyridines (nifedipine, felodipine) but may occur with any calcium channel blocker

   i. Effect lessened when used in combination with ACE inhibitor

   ii. Due to change in transcapillary pressure in extremities and should **not** be treated with increased diuresis

  d. Less effective as second drug added to diuretic

  e. Potentially serious limiting side effects (see Table 11)

   i. Dihydropyridines: orthostasis and tachycardia

   ii. Diltiazem and verapamil: atrioventricular block

   iii. Most have some negative inotropic effect: verapamil > diltiazem > nifedipine/nicardipine

TABLE II. Comparison of Incidence of Problems with Calcium Channel Blockers

Problems	Verapamil > Diltiazem	Dihydropyridines
Orthostasis	Low	Moderate
Use with beta blockers or in presence of atrioventricular block	No	Yes
Negative inotropic effects	Moderate	Low
Tachycardia	No	Moderate to high
Constipation	Moderate	Low
Edema	Low	High

    iv. Differences in cardiovascular and renal outcomes between two major subclasses of calcium channel blockers currently available (see Table 12)

3. **Safety and efficacy**

    a. Retrospective studies support concept that **short-acting** calcium channel blockers in moderate-to-high doses adversely affect cardiovascular outcomes

    b. In high-risk populations (i.e., diabetics with hypertension and renal disease), long-acting dihydropyridines do not reduce risk of cardiovascular events despite blood pressure reduction. Conversely, nondihydropyridines reduce renal disease progression and proteinuria; moreover, they are the only calcium channel blockers shown to reduce mortality from ischemic heart disease

    c. Several studies suggest that calcium channel blockers are probably safe in patients with angina, patients who have suffered myocardial infarction, hypertensive patients with coronary disease, and elderly hypertensives. Only short-acting dihydropyridines have demonstrated possible increase in cardiovascular mortality associated with ischemic disease. The combination of a dihydropyridine calcium channel blocker with an ACE inhibitor has been shown to reduce cardiovascular risk to levels comparable to that of ACE inhibitors alone. Moreover, this combination is well tolerated and has lower side-effect profile

    d. Nondihydropyridines are superior to beta blockers for slowing progression of diabetic nephropathy. Some studies suggest that they may have efficacy comparable to ACE inhibitors in curtailing progression of diabetic renal disease[34,35]

    e. SYST-EUR study[36] confirmed clear reduction in cardiovascular mortality in elderly patients with hypertension treated with nitrendipine. The study, however, used a true placebo that did not control blood pressure. Thus, another conclusion from this study is that blood pressure control, regardless of agent used, reduces cardiovascular events

    f. Taken together, studies demonstrate that long-acting dihydropyridines are effective antihypertensive agents. They may not, however, provide maximal cardiovascular protection in at-risk people with pre-existing target-organ injury, such as those with renal insufficiency and diabetes. However, combination of ACE inhibitor and dihydropyridine has been shown to reduce cardiovascular risk to levels comparable to that of ACE inhibitors alone. Moreover, this combination is well tolerated and has lower side-effect profile

TABLE 12. Summary of Calcium Antagonist Controversy

		CV Mortality	Renal Disease Progression
DHP CCBs	Short-acting	↑	??
	Long-acting	→ ↓ *	→
nonDHP CCBs	Short-acting	→	? ↓
	Long-acting	↓	↓

* Nitrendipine in Syst-Eur trial. ↑ = increase, ↓ = decrease, → = no effect.

G. **Combined beta and alpha blockers**
   1. Combined alpha-1/nonselective beta blocker with beta-2 ISA:labetalol
      a. Potent
      b. High incidence of postural hypotension
      c. Contraindications same as beta blockers
      d. Fatigue and impotence common
      e. Alpha:beta activity in 1:3 (oral) to 1:7 (parenteral) ratio
      f. Does not lower HDL
      g. May not be cardioprotective after myocardial infarction
   2. Combined alpha-1 and nonselective beta blocker without ISA: carvedilol
      a. Approved for treatment of hypertension and congestive heart failure (CHF) even in absence of hypertension
      b. Usage in CHF often complicated despite major potential benefit[37]
         i. Patients may worsen for several months
         ii. Lower starting dosages than with hypertension
         iii. Cardiology consultation recommended for patients with class II, III, or IV CHF

H. **Fixed-dose combinations**
   1. Multiple combinations available (see Appendix V Supplement)
   2. Not approved by FDA for initial therapy with following exceptions
      a. Bisoprolol/hydrochlorothiazide (Ziac)[38]
      b. Captopril/hydrochlorothiazide (Capozide)
   3. **Advantages**
      a. May reduce cost (usually less expensive than components purchased separately)
      b. Usually lower side-effect profile than either drug alone[23]
      c. Usually improve compliance
      d. Combined effects may have greater benefit than either drug alone
         i. Nondihydropyridines with ACE inhibitors more effectively reduce proteinuria and slow progression of renal disease than either drug alone
         ii. ACE inhibitors may reduce risk of diuretic-associated hypokalemia
         iii. ACE inhibitors reduce edema from calcium channel blockers
         iv. Diuretics lessen tendency to develop hyperkalemia in patients taking ACE inhibitors
         v. Some diuretic/beta blocker and ACE inhibitor/calcium channel blocker combinations have been shown to result in fewer side effects and yet have greater efficacy than either drug alone[23,39,40]

4. Low-dose combinations considered acceptable as second-line treatment and should be considered for initial therapy with stage II or III hypertension[41]

IV. **Approach to Therapy**

A. **Customized therapy:** rather than using "cookbook" approach, we favor development of "antihypertensive cocktail" individualized for each patient and his or her associated medical conditions[42]

1. **General and constitutional characteristics** are easily derived from JNC VI. We extend these recommendations to specific issues not discussed in JNC VI

   a. **Noncompliant or "no-show" patients**
      i. Calcium channel blockers (once-daily formulations)
      ii. Low-dose diuretics
      iii. Selective alpha-1 blockers (alternative)

   b. **Patients with anxiety or insomnia**
      i. Beta blockers
      ii. Central alpha-2 agonists

   c. **Patients with orthostasis** (*not* together)
      i. Clonidine *or*
      ii. Beta blockers

   d. **Young persons**
      i. ACE inhibitors (**absolutely contraindicated** in women who may become pregnant)
      ii. Calcium channel blockers
      iii. Low-dose thiazide diuretics

   e. **Young and "hyperdynamic" persons**
      i. Verapamil
      ii. Beta blockers without ISA

   f. **Patients who exercise**
      i. ACE inhibitors
      ii. Alpha-1 blockers
      iii. Calcium channel blockers
      iv. Central agents other than methyldopa
      v. Avoid non-ISA beta blockers
      vi. Angiotensin II receptor blockers

   g. **Elderly patients (especially with ISH)**
      i. Diuretics (preferred)
      ii. Calcium channel blockers (long-acting)
      iii. ACE inhibitors
      iv. Nitrates (especially with history of coronary artery disease)[43]

   h. **African-Americans**
      i. Diuretics
      ii. Calcium channel blockers
      iii. Angiotensin receptor blockers
         (a) Trandolapril approved as first-line therapy by FDA
         (b) Candesartan and valsartan also effective
      iv. Labetalol (monitor liver function tests; stop drug if abnormal)
      v. ACE inhibitors in moderate-to-high doses (higher incidence of angioedema than in other patients)

   i. **Obese patients**
      i. Diuretics
      ii. Calcium channel blockers

j. **Young women intending to have children**
  i. Avoid ACE inhibitors and angiotensin II blockers
  ii. Methyldopa (preferred)
  iii. Atenolol, metoprolol—**not** with methyldopa

k. **Impotent patients**
  i. ACE inhibitors
  ii. Angiotensin-II receptor blockers
  iii. Alpha-1 blockers
  iv. Calcium channel blockers
  v. Avoid beta blockers, central agents, and diuretics

l. **Women with menopausal symptoms**
  i. Central alpha-2 agonists
  ii. Avoid dihydropyridine calcium channel blockers

m. **Patients with depression**
  i. ACE inhibitors
  ii. Angiotensin-II receptor blockers
  iii. Alpha-1 blockers
  iv. Calcium channel blockers
  v. Avoid methyldopa, reserpine, and beta blockers
  vi. In affective disorders, monoamine oxidase (MAO) inhibitors are said to be effective in treating both depression and hypertension

n. **Patients with rhinitis and sinusitis**
  i. Central alpha-2 agonists
  ii. Avoid beta blockers, reserpine, and alpha blockers

o. **Patients with arthritis** (50% of patients over 65 have osteoarthritic changes on radiograph[44])
  i. Calcium channel blockers
  ii. Alpha blockers
  iii. Use ACE inhibitors or angiotensin-II blockers **with caution** in patients taking NSAIDs or those with elevated creatinine
    (a) NSAIDs may antagonize these drugs
    (b) Hyperkalemia is more likely when these drugs are used together in patients with elevated creatinine, especially diabetics
  iv. Avoid NSAIDs in hypertensive patients with renal insufficiency if at all possible (worsen hypertension)
  v. Nonacetylated (non–aspirin-like) salicylates, such as salsalate (Disalcid) and choline magnesium trisalicylate (Trilisate), may be least likely to interact with antihypertensive medications
  vi. Among traditional nonsteroidal agents, sulindac (Clinoril) seems to interact least often; naproxen also may be less likely to interact. Most others antagonize antihypertensives
  vii. Coadministration of potassium-sparing diuretics and beta blockers as well as ACE inhibitors results in higher incidence of hyperkalemia with NSAIDs. Close monitoring of potassium and creatinine is mandatory when any of these is combined with NSAID. Generally, use of potassium-sparing diuretics together with ACE inhibitor is contraindicated

2. **Special forms of hypertension** (see also Chapter 5)
   a. **Spinal cord dysreflexia syndrome** (see also Chapter 2)
      i. Nonselective alpha blockers
      ii. Calcium channel blockers
      iii. Nitrates
      iv. Nitroprusside
      v. Avoid central alpha agonists
   b. **Baroreflex failure syndrome** [45] (see also Chapter 2)
      i. For anxiety-precipitated attacks, use benzodiazepine
      ii. Clonidine (patch or tablets in high dosage)
      iii. Phenoxybenzamine (up to 100 mg/day)
      iv. Early in course avoid mental stress
3. **Organ dysfunction**
   a. **Neurologic disorders**
      i. **Migraine**
         (a) Beta blockers
         (b) Calcium channel blockers (verapamil preferred)
         (c) Central nervous system-acting agents
      ii. **Essential tremor:** beta blockers
      iii. **Cerebrovascular disease** (**not** acute stroke; acute hypertension from ischemic stroke generally should be treated with extreme caution if at all; see pages 17 and 70). In all cases, postural hypotension must be avoided. Potentially advantageous drugs may include
         (a) Calcium channel blockers
         (b) ACE inhibitors
         (c) Low-dose thiazide diuretics
         (d) Beta blockers or central alpha agonists—only with postural hypotension or centrally mediated hypertension (may cause CNS depression)
   b. **Cardiovascular conditions**
      i. **After myocardial infarction**
         (a) Beta blockers without ISA have proven efficacy in lowering mortality rate
         (b) Heart rate-lowering calcium channel blockers (verapamil, diltiazem) also have shown efficacy in reducing mortality rate[46–49]
         (c) ACE inhibitors have been shown to improve outcome in patients with left ventricular dysfunction, even when dysfunction is asymptomatic[37]
      ii. **Supraventricular tachycardias or angina**
         (a) Beta blockers
         (b) Heart rate-lowering calcium channel blockers
      iii. **Bradycardia:** direct vasodilators
      iv. **Left ventricular hypertrophy**[50–55]
         (a) ACE inhibitors[32,33] may be most effective
         (b) Nondihydropyridine calcium channel blockers[32,33]
         (c) Beta blockers
         (d) Diuretics[34]
      v. **Congestive heart failure** (CHF)
         (a) Diuretics

    (b) ACE inhibitors
- (i) Use cautiously; avoid NSAIDs
- (ii) Prolong survival in patients with CHF[56–59]

    (c) Angiotensin II receptor blockers: preliminary data suggest that losartan is at least as effective as captopril in patients with CHF and ejection fraction below 40%[60]

  vi. **Coarctation of aorta**
- (a) Preoperative management: ACE inhibitors or beta blockers
- (b) Postsurgical hypertension[61]: prevention with beta blockers and/or ACE inhibitors
- (c) Late exercise-induced hypertension[62]: alpha blockers and other traditional agents

c. **Pulmonary conditions**

  i. **Asthma and chronic obstructive pulmonary disease** (COPD)
- (a) Calcium channel blockers preferred[63,64]
- (b) Beta blockers of all types contraindicated except beta-1 selective agents, which may be used **cautiously if necessary and in low doses** in patients who have COPD but **no history of bronchospasm**
- (c) Use of following is possible in low doses and with caution
  - (i) Central alpha-2 agonists and alpha-1 blockers may increase subjective dyspnea or increase sensitivity to histamine[65,66]
  - (ii) Diuretics
    - Hypokalemia is additive to that induced by inhaled or oral beta agonists and steroids
    - Metabolic alkalosis may reduce hypoxic drive in patients with severe COPD
    - In patients taking theophylline preparations, tendency to arrhythmias and seizures is likely to be enhanced by hypokalemia or alkalosis
  - (iii) ACE inhibitors
    - Avoid in asthma especially[67]
    - May be beneficial in pulmonary hypertension
  - (iv) Angiotensin receptor blockers: no apparent contraindications at time of this writing

  ii. **Pulmonary hypertension**
- (a) Calcium channel blockers (preferred)
  - (i) Especially long-acting dihydropyridines
  - (ii) High doses recommended
- (b) ACE inhibitors may be beneficial in some patients
- (c) Thromboxane synthetase inhibitors and prostaglandin analogs also have shown some promise

d. **Gastrointestinal conditions**

  i. **Peptic ulcer disease:** avoid reserpine, ganglionic blockers

  ii. **Liver disease**
- (a) Use
  - (i) Alpha-1 blockers
  - (ii) Diuretics (with caution if patient has ascites)

(iii) Nonselective beta blockers (with varices)

(iv) ACE inhibitors may be used with caution, but avoid use of NSAIDs

(v) No apparent contraindication to angiotensin II receptor blockers

(b) Avoid

(i) Labetalol

(ii) Methyldopa

e. **Renal and genitourinary disorders**

i. **Renal impairment**[68,69] (see also Appendix VI)

(a) In most cases, sodium restriction to 2–3 gm/day (5–8 gm NaCl or about 85–120 mEq sodium) is necessary for optimal blood pressure control.[5] In **very rare circumstances** some patients are actually volume-depleted due to salt wasting; their hypertension is worsened by salt restriction[69]

(b) Rigorous control of hypertension is critical to minimize progression of renal disease. Analysis of data from recent study that looked at effect of protein restriction on progression of renal disease revealed dramatic effect of blood pressure control on delaying progression of renal disease[27,28] (Fig. 7)

(c) Goal of therapy is blood pressure ≤ 130/85 mmHg[5,70] in anyone with

(i) Over 1 gm/day of proteinuria and/or

(ii) Renal insufficiency and/or

(iii) Diabetes mellitus

(d) African-Americans also may require blood pressure ≤ 130/85 mmHg to delay deterioration of renal function[5,71]

(e) Effect of low-protein diets[70]

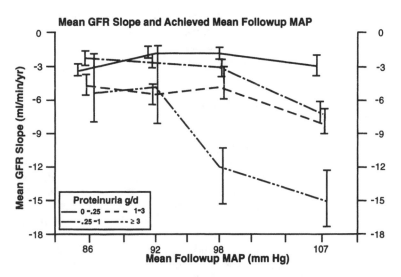

FIGURE 7. Mean glomerular filtration rate (GFR) slope and achieved mean follow-up arterial pressure. (Baseline GFR is 25–55 ml/min.)

(i) Modest protein restriction to 0.6 gm/kg/day seems to have some (albeit limited) effect in slowing progression of renal impairment; more severe restriction has shown little or no advantage[70]

(ii) Modification of Diet in Renal Disease (MDRD) study showed much more dramatic effect of blood pressure reduction, which was far greater than effect of diet[70]

(f) **Drugs of value**

  (i) Loop diuretics
- Most important drug in control of hypertension that is of renal parenchymal origin
- Few patients with azotemia have hypertension that is controllable unless diuretics are part of treatment

  (ii) Calcium channel blockers

  (iii) Central agents

  (iv) ACE inhibitors
- Up to serum creatinine of about 3.5 mg/dl or creatinine clearance > about 35 cc/min
- Reduce doses by 50% or use drugs not metabolized or excreted by kidney (fosinopril, ramipril, trandolapril)

  (v) Angiotensin II receptor blockers
- Good antihypertensive agents
- Trials in patients with renal disease pending

  (vi) ACE inhibitors with calcium channel blockers (preferred)[71–72]

  (vii) Occasional patients require therapy with minoxidil,[73] which in turn requires simultaneous use of diuretic and sympathetic inhibitor, such as beta blocker or central alpha agonist

  (viii) Combined calcium antagonists of two different classes (e.g., diltiazem or verapamil plus nifedipine XL) also may be effective in resistant cases[74]

(g) **Effects of NSAIDs on hypertension in renal disease**

  (i) Many antagonize most antihypertensive agents, including beta blockers and diuretics,[75–81] but not calcium channel blockers[82]

  (ii) May interfere with vasodilatory prostaglandins and reduce renal perfusion

  (iii) Dramatically increase risk of hyperkalemia when given with ACE inhibitors in azotemic patients; effect on antihypertensive effects of ACE inhibitors is not well established

  (iv) Risk of worsening renal function and acute renal failure when coadministered with ACE inhibitor[83,84]

  (v) Sulindac and low-dose aspirin may be less likely to reduce antihypertensive drug effectiveness than other NSAIDs; sulindac may still interact with labetalol

ii. **Renal artery stenosis**

(a) Calcium channel blockers

(b) Beta blockers

    (c) Minoxidil in resistant cases

    (d) ACE inhibitors or angiotensin II receptor blockers may be useful with unilateral renal artery stenosis

    (e) Avoid use of ACE inhibitors in patients with bilateral stenosis, stenosis in solitary kidney, or stenosis in renal transplant

  iii. **Nephrolithiasis due to hypercalciuria** (most kidney stones): thiazides

  iv. **After renal transplant**

    (a) Calcium channel blockers

      (i) With dihydropyridines, generally no cyclosporine dose adjustment is needed (except amlodipine)

      (ii) With verapamil and diltiazem, reduce cyclosporine dose

      (iii) Reduced incidence of acute tubular necrosis and rejection with verapamil[85]

    (b) Central agents

    (c) Labetalol

  v. **Prostatic hypertrophy:** once-daily alpha-1 blockers

f. **Sickle cell disease**[86]

  i. Patients usually have lower blood pressure than normal

  ii. Mild elevations of blood pressure may dramatically increase risk to greater extent than in patients without underlying disease

  iii. Although no prospective data exist about treatment, it seems prudent to maintain blood pressure in optimal range

  iv. Avoid volume depletion or diuretics, which may precipitate crises

g. **Endocrine and metabolic disorders**

  i. **Hyperlipidemia**

    (a) Alpha blockers   (d) Indapamide

    (b) Calcium blockers   (e) Beta blockers with ISA

    (c) ACE inhibitors

  ii. **Early diabetes mellitus** (microalbuminuria without azotemia)

    (a) ACE inhibitors alone (with monitoring of potassium)—proven to slow progression (preferred)

      (i) Delay progression in type I diabetes mellitus, even in normotensive patients with isolated microalbuminuria[87,88]

      (ii) Slow progression of established renal disease in patients with type I diabetes mellitus[29]

      (iii) Effective in slowing progression of both azotemia and microalbuminuria in hypertensive patients with type II diabetes mellitus when added to effective control of blood pressure despite no significant further drop in blood pressure[89]

      (iv) Also shown to be effective in slowing progression of nephropathy in normotensive type II diabetes[90]

    (b) ACE inhibitors with calcium channel blockers added

      (i) Only for coronary disease or difficult-to-control hypertension

      (ii) Nondihydropyridine types preferred[21,22,91]

  (iii) Although addition of nondihydropyridines to ACE inhibitors reduces proteinuria further, it is currently unknown whether this has beneficial long-term effect on human renal function. Recent animal study showed that ACE inhibitors or combination of ACE inhibitors and nondihydropyridines prevented mesangial expansion[46]

(c) ACE inhibitors with diuretics—for difficult-to-control hypertension with sodium retention due to
 (i) Congestive heart failure
 (ii) Edema due to renal failure or nephrotic syndrome

(d) Alpha blockers also may be used without adverse effects but have not been shown to have potential benefit of other regimens on preservation of renal function

(e) When beta blockers are required, beta-1 selective agents in lowest possible doses should be used
 (i) Addition makes hyperkalemia more likely
 (ii) Because in overt nephropathy beta blockers are inferior to ACE inhibitors and nondihydropyridines,[34] it may be prudent to avoid them in any stage of diabetes mellitus unless specific indication supports their use
 (iii) Sometimes required (e.g., after myocardial infarction, with angina)

iii. **Late diabetes mellitus** (serum creatinine ≥ 1.5 mg/dl and proteinuria > 1 gm/24 hr)

(a) Aggressive control of hypertension (< 130 systolic and < 85 diastolic) is critically important in delaying progressive renal deterioration of overt diabetic nephropathy[92]

(b) Diuretics almost always required to control blood pressure

(c) ACE inhibitors (in reduced dosage) and/or nondihydropyridine calcium channel blockers[34]

(d) Evidence suggests that once proteinuria or azotemia is established, ACE inhibitors may still slow progression of renal disease

(e) Close monitoring of creatinine and potassium as well as magnitude of proteinuria is required

(f) Recent data suggest that antihypertensive agents that blunt rise in proteinuria over time preserve renal function to greater extent than agents without such effects.[20–22,25,26] This may apply even in absence of changes in blood pressure.[19] Primary agents are ACE inhibitors and nondihydropyridines

(g) One recent small study supported the notion that in azotemic patients with frank proteinuria, a low-protein, low-phosphorus diet might delay progression of diabetic nephropathy[93]

iv. **Pheochromocytoma** (see Appendix III for perioperative management)

(a) Medical management is necessary until surgery and during pregnancy; also required in patients with metastatic malignant pheochromocytoma[94]

(b) Drug therapy

(i) Nonselective alpha blockers are mainstay of therapy; phenoxybenzamine, 10–20 mg 4 times/day, and titrated to control pressure

(ii) Peripheral alpha-2 blockers such as prazosin also have been used

(iii) Calcium channel blockers have theoretical advantages of avoiding postural hypotension and overshoot hypotension

(iv) Beta blockers also may be needed in patients with disproportionate beta-1 (epinephrine-like) activity
- **Contraindicated until** patient is well alpha-blocked, because beta-2 agonist activity of the secreted hormone produces vasodilation and antagonizes vasoconstrictive alpha-1 effects
- If beta blockade alone is used, hypertension may worsen dramatically

(v) During surgery
- Nitroprusside and/or phentolamine are used parenterally
- Short-acting beta blocker esmolol may be **added**, if necessary, to control cardiac arrhythmias, although lidocaine also has been used

v. **Hyperaldosteronism**
  (a) Solitary tumors are usually resected
  (b) Drug therapy
    (i) In bilateral adrenal hyperplasia, spironolactone is drug of choice (up to 400 mg/day)[94]
    (ii) Amiloride (up to 40 mg/day) may be used in place of spironolactone to lessen side effects, particularly in men
    (iii) Triamterene is **not** as effective but may be tried in patients intolerant of spironolactone and amiloride
    (iv) In many cases thiazide diuretics need to be added (12.5–25 mg hydrochlorothiazide daily)
    (v) Some patients may need addition of third drug
      - Calcium channel blockers and ACE inhibitors have been suggested as effective options
      - In patients with bilateral adrenal hyperplasia, combinations of spironolactone, 300 mg/day, with fixed-dose combination of ACE inhibitor/calcium channel blocker achieved blood pressure control to < 140/90 in all subjects
    (vi) In all cases, careful monitoring of serum potassium during therapy is needed
  (c) Postoperative **hypo**aldosteronism may occur
    (i) **Potassium must be monitored after surgery**
    (ii) Potassium should be administered with great caution
  (d) **Adrenogenital syndrome and glucocorticoid-responsive hyperaldosteronism** (see Appendix II)
    (i) Treat with low-dose prednisone (e.g., 5–7.5 mg/day)
    (ii) Occasional patients may require slightly higher doses
    (iii) Patients require increased doses during stress

B. **Without coexisting diseases or conditions listed above** (Fig. 8)

Salt restriction (2 gm sodium = 80 mEq Na), weight loss, exercise,
reduction of tobacco, reduction of alcohol

↓ Pressure remains elevated

Start low-dose and long-acting thiazide, beta blocker, calcium channel blocker, low-dose
ACE inhibitor, angiotensin-II receptor blocker, or peripheral alpha-1 blocker

↓ Pressure remains elevated

Double initial dosage, substitute another drug, or consider low-dose combination drug

↓ Pressure remains elevated

Add low-dose thiazide or substitute another drug

↓ Pressure remains elevated

Full dose of current drug

↓ Pressure remains elevated

Reevaluate:
Compliance with diet or medications
Secondary causes
Intraarterial blood pressure, especially in elderly
Ambulatory blood pressure monitoring

↓ Pressure remains elevated

Add ACE inhibitor or angiotensin-II blocker if not already used

(caution in patients taking diuretics)

↓ Pressure remains elevated

Add calcium channel blocker if not already used

↓ Pressure remains elevated

Add appropriate drug from another class, such as:
Clonidine
Hydralazine
Beta blocker (caution with calcium channel blockers)

↓ Pressure remains elevated

Add minoxidil, withdraw all medications except

beta blocker or clonidine and loop diuretic

↓ Pressure remains elevated

Strongly consider either noncompliance or secondary cause

FIGURE 8. Approach to blood pressure reduction in uncomplicated hypertensive patients. In patients with stage I hypertension, if the initial choice fails, substituting a drug of a different class is preferable to adding another drug, because only about 50% of patients respond to any given choice. Sequential substitution results in control of 75% of patients by the third drug substitution.[95] In patients with stage 2 or 3 hypertension, an average of about 4 (3.2–4.5) different antihypertensive medications is required to achieve adequate control; fixed-dose combinations should be considered strongly as second-line therapy to improve compliance and maintain blood pressure control.[96]

C. **Be aware of potential side effects** (see Appendix VII). Sensitivity by physician to benign yet annoying side effects increases compliance

D. **Monitor appropriate parameters** when using drugs with potentially serious side effects

1. **Potassium**
   a. ACE inhibitors
   b. Diuretics
   c. Beta blockers (in diabetic or azotemic patients)

2. **Liver function**
   a. Labetalol
   b. Methyldopa
   c. Hydralazine

3. **Blood counts**
   a. ACE inhibitors
   b. Methyldopa
   c. Hydralazine
   d. Diuretics
   e. Minoxidil

4. **Renal function** should be monitored in all hypertensive patients but is particularly important in
   a. All diabetics
   b. All patients taking beta blockers
   c. All patients taking ACE inhibitors
   d. All patients taking diuretics

REFERENCES

1. Powers WJ: Acute hypertension after stroke: The scientific basis for treatment decisions. Neurology 1993;43:461–467.
2. SHEP Cooperative Research Group: Prevention of stroke by antihypertensive drug treatment in older patients with isolated systolic hypertension: Final results of the Systolic Hypertension in the Elderly Program (SHEP). JAMA 1991;265:3255–3264.
3. Staessen JA, Fagard R, et al: Randomized double-blind placebo and active treatment for older patients with isolated systolic hypertension (Syst-Eur Trial). Lancet 1997;350: 757–764.
4. Michelis MF: Systolic hypertension in the elderly: Reasons not to treat. Am J Kidney Dis 1990;16:332–334.
5. Sixth Report of the Joint National Committee on Detection, Evaluation and Treatment of High Blood Pressure (JNC VI). Arch Intern Med 1997;157:2413–2445.
6. Grin JM, McCabe EJ, White WB: Management of hypertension after ambulatory blood pressure monitoring. Ann Intern Med 1993;118:833–837.
7. Zachariah PK, Sheps SG, Bailey KR, et al: Age-related characteristics of ambulatory blood pressure load and mean blood pressure in normal subjects. JAMA 1991;265: 1414–1417.
8. Peterson JC, Adler S, et al: Blood pressure control, proteinuria, and the progression of renal disease. The Modification of Diet in Renal Disease Study. Ann Intern Med 1995;123:754–762.
9. Lazarus JM, Bourgoine JJ, Buckalew VM, et al: Achievement and safety of a lower blood pressure goal in chronic renal disease: The Modification of Diet in Renal Disease Study Group. Hypertension 1997;29:641–650.
10. Krumholz HM, Parent EM, et al: Readmission after hospitalization for congestive heart failure among Medicare beneficiaries. Arch Intern Med 1997;157:99–104.
11. Du X, Cruickshank K, et al: Case control study of stroke and the quality of hypertension control in northwest England. BMJ 1997;314:272–276.

12. Hansson L, Zanchetti A, Carruthers SG, et al: Effects of intensive blood pressure lowering and low-dose aspirin in patients with hypertension: Principal results of the Hypertension Optimal Treatment (HOT) randomised trial. HOT Study Group. Lancet 1998;351:1755–1762.
13. Weinberger MH: Influence of an angiotensin converting-enzyme inhibitor on diuretic-induced metabolic effects in hypertension. Hypertension 1983;5:132–138.
14. Bakris GL, Smith A: Effects of sodium intake on albumin excretion in patients with diabetic nephropathy in patients treated with long-acting calcium antagonists. Ann Intern Med 1996;124:201–204.
15. Bakris GL, Mehler PS, Schrier RW: Hypertension and diabetes. In Schrier RW, Gottschalk CW (eds): Diseases of the Kidney, 6th ed. Boston, Little, Brown, 1996, pp 1455–1464.
16. Preston RA, Singer I, Epstein M: Renal parenchymal hypertension: Current concepts of pathogenesis and management. Arch Intern Med 1996;156:602–611.
17. Linas SL: The role of potassium in the pathogenesis of hypertension. Kidney Int 1991;39:771–786.
18. Khaw KT, Barrett-Conner E: Dietary potassium and stroke related mortality: A 12-year prospective population study. N Engl J Med 1987;316:236–240.
19. Siani A, Strazzullo P, Giacco A, et al: Increasing the dietary potassium intake reduces the need for antihypertensive medication. Ann Intern Med 1991;115:753–759.
20. Le QT, Elliott WJ: Dose-response relationship of blood pressure and serum cholesterol to 3-n-butyl phthalide, a component of celery oil. Clin Res 1991;39:750A.
21. Le QT, Elliott WJ: Mechanisms of the hypotensive effect of 3-n-butyl phthalide, a component of celery oil. Clin Res 1992;40:326A.
22. Papademetriou V, Fletcher R, Khatri IM, Freis ED: Diuretic-induced hypokalemia in uncomplicated systemic hypertension: Effect of plasma potassium correction on cardiac arrhythmias. Am J Cardiol 1983;52:1017–1022.
23. Papademetriou V: Diuretics, hypokalemia and cardiac arrhythmias: A critical analysis. Am Heart J 1986;111:1217–1224.
24. Caralis PV, Materson BJ, Perez-Stable E: Potassium and diuretic-induced ventricular arrhythmias in ambulatory hypertensive patients. Miner Electrolyte Metab 1984;10:148–154.
25. Freis ED: Thiazide diuretics: How real are the concerns? [editorial]. Hosp Pract 1990;25:8–14.
26. Madias JE, Madias NE: Dose diuretic-induced hypokalemia cause ventricular arrhythmias? Primary Cardiol 1987;8:31–41.
27. DeFronzo RA, Bonadonna RC, Ferrannini E: Pathogenesis of NIDDM: A balanced overview. Diabetic Care 1992;15:318–368.
28. Toto RD, Mitchell HC, Lee H, et al: Reversible renal insufficiency due to angiotensin converting enzyme inhibitors in hypertensive nephrosclerosis. Ann Intern Med 1991;115:513–519.
29. Lewis EJ, Hunsicker LG, Bain RP, et al: The effects of angiotensin converting enzyme inhibition in diabetic nephropathy. N Engl J Med 1993;329:1456–1462.
30. Slataper R, Vicknair R, Sadler R, et al: Comparative effects of different antihypertensive treatments on progression of diabetic renal disease. Arch Intern Med 1993;153:973–980.
31. Bakris GL, Barnhill BW, Sadler R: Treatment of arterial hypertension in diabetic humans: Importance of therapeutic selection. Kidney Int 1992;41:912–919.
32. Brown SA, Walton CL, Crawford P, et al: Long term effects of antihypertensive regimens on renal hemodynamics and proteinuria. Kidney Int 1993;43:1210–1218.
33. Pitt B, Segal R, et al: Randomised trial of losartan versus captopril in patients over 65 with heart failure (Evaluation of Losartan in the Elderly Study ELITE). Lancet 1997;349:747–752.
34. Bakris GL, Copley JB, et al: Calcium channel blockers versus other antihypertensive therapies on progression of NIDDM associated nephropathy. Kidney Int 1996;50:1641–1650.
35. Bakris GL, Mangrum A, et al: Effect of calcium channel or beta-blockade on the the progression of diabetic nephropathy in African-Americans. AHA Hypertens 1997;29:745–750.
36. Staessen JA, Fagard R, Thijs L, et al: Randomised double-blind comparison of placebo and active treatment for older patients with isolated systolic hypertension. The Systolic Hypertension in Europe (Sys-Eur) Trial Investigators. Lancet 1997;350:757–764.

37. Packer M, Bristow MR, et al: The effect of carvedilol on morbidity and mortality in patients with chronic heart failure. U.S. Carvedilol Heart Failure Study Group. N Engl J Med 1996;334:1349–1355.

38. Prisant JM, Weir MR, et al: Low dose drug combination therapy: An alternative first line approach to hypertensive treatment. Am Heart J 1995;130:359–366.

39. Gradman AH, Cutler NR, Davis PJ, et al: Combined enalapril and felodipine extended release (ER) for systemic hypertension. Am J Cardiol 1997;79:431–435.

40. Morgan TO, Anderson A, Jones E: Comparison and interaction of low dose felodipine and enalapril in the treatment of essential hypertension in elderly patients. Am J Hypertens 1992;5:238–243.

41. Esptein M, Bakris G: Newer approaches to antihypertensive therapy. Arch Intern Med 1996;156:1969–1978.

42. Houston M: New insights and approaches to reduce end-organ damage in the treatment of hypertension: Subsets of hypertension approach. Am Heart J 1992;123:1337–1367.

43. Duchier J, Iannascoli F, Safar M: Antihypertensive effect of sustained release isosorbide dinitrate for isolated systolic hypertension in the elderly. Am J Cardiol 1987;60:99.

44. Peyron JG: Epidemiologic and etiologic approach to osteoarthritis. Semin Arthritis Rheum 1979;8:288–306.

45. Robertson D, Hollister AS, Biaggioni I, et al: The diagnosis and therapy of baroreflex failure. N Engl J Med 1993;329:1449–1455.

46. Gibson RS, Boden WE, Theroux P, et al: Diltiazem and reinfarction in patients with non-q wave myocardial infarction: Results of a double blind, randomized, multicenter trial. N Engl J Med 1986;315:423–429.

47. Gibson RS: Current status of calcium channel blocking drugs after q wave and non-q wave myocardial infarction. Circulation 1989;80:107–119.

48. Danish Study Group on Verapamil in Myocardial Infarction: Effect of verapamil on mortality and major events after acute myocardial infarction. Am J Cardiol 1990;66: 799–810.

49. Pepine CJ: Pharmacotherapy of myocardial infarction: Current perspectives. In Epstein M (ed): Calcium antagonists in Clinical Medicine. Philadelphia, Hanley & Belfus, 1992, pp 165–182.

50. Frohlich ED, Apstein C, Chobanian AV, et al: The heart in hypertension. N Engl J Med 1992;327:998.

51. Dahlof B, Pennert K, Hansson L: Reversal of left ventricular hypertrophy in hypertensive patients: A meta-analysis of 109 treatment studies. Am J Hypertens 1992;5:95.

52. Schulman SP, Weiss JL, Becker LC, et al: The effects of antihypertensive therapy on left ventricular mass in elderly patients. N Engl J Med 1990;322:1350–1356.

53. Frohlich ED, Horinaka S: Cardiac and aortic effects of angiotensin converting enzyme inhibitors. Hypertension 1991;18(Suppl II):II2–II7.

54. Frohlich ED: Left ventricular hypertrophy, cardiac diseases and hypertension. In Knoebel SB, Dack S (eds): An Era in Cardiovascular Medicine. New York, Elsevier, 1991, pp 85–92.

55. Neaton JD, Grimm RH, Prineas RJ, et al: Treatment of mild hypertension study: Final results. JAMA 1993;270:713–724.

56. Pfeiffer MA, Braunwald E, Moge LA, et al: Effect of captopril on mortality and morbidity in patients with left ventricular dysfunction after myocardial infarction: Results of the survival and ventricular enlargement trial. N Engl J Med 1992;327:669.

57. Cohn JN, Johnson G, Ziesche S, et al: A comparison of enalapril with hydralazine-isosorbide dinitrate in the treatment of chronic congestive heart failure. N Engl J Med 1991;325:303.

58. SOLVD Investigators: Effect of enalapril on mortality and morbidity and the development of heart failure in asymptomatic patients with reduced left ventricular ejection fractions. N Engl J Med 1992;327:685.

59. SOLVD Investigators: Effect of enalapril on survival in patients with reduced left ventricular ejection fractions and congestive heart failure. N Engl J Med 1991;325:293.

60. Gidding SS, Rocchini AP, Beekman R, et al: Therapeutic effect of propranolol on paradoxical hypertension after repair of coarctation of the aorta. N Engl J Med 1985;312: 1224–1228.

61. Markel H, Rocchini AP, Beekman R, et al: Exercise-induced hypertension after repair of coarctation of the aorta: Arm versus leg exercise. J Am Coll Cardiol 1986;8:165–171.

62. Barnes PJ: Clinical studies with calcium antagonists in asthma. Br J Clin Pharmacol 1985;20:289s.

63. Schwartzstein RS, Fanta CH: Orally administered nifedipine in chronic stable asthma: Comparison with an orally administered sympathomimetic. Am Rev Respir Dis 1986;79:959.

64. Dinh AT, Matran R, et al: Comparative effects of rilmenidine and clonidine on bronchial responses to histamine in asthmatic patients. Br J Clin Pharmacol 1988;26:703.

65. Chodosh S, Tuck J, Pizzuto D: Prazosin in hypertensive patients with chronic bronchitis and asthma: A brief report. Am J Med 1989;86:91.

66. Lipworth BJ, McMurray JJ, Clark RA, Struthers AD: Development of late onset asthma following treatment with captopril. Eur Respir J 1989;2:586.

67. Preston RA, Singer I, Epstein M: Renal parenchymal hypertension: Current concepts of pathogenesis and management. Arch Intern Med 1996;156:602–611.

68. National High Blood Pressure Education Program Working Group: 1995 Update of the Working Group Reports on Chronic Renal Failure and Renovascular Hypertension. Arch Intern Med 1996;156:1938–1947.

69. Uribarri J, Oh MS, Carrl HJ: Salt-losing nephropathy: Clinical presentations and mechanisms. Am J Nephrol 1983;3:193–198.

70. Klahr S, Levey AS, Beck GJ, et al: The effects of dietary protein restriction and blood pressure control on the progression of chronic renal disease. N Engl J Med 1994;330: 877–885.

71. Tolins JP, Raij L: Antihypertensive therapy and the progression of renal disease. Semin Nephrol 1991;11:538–548.

72. Wenzel UO, Helmchen U, et al: Combination treatment of enalapril with nitrendipine in rats with renovascular hypertension. Hypertension 1994;23:114–122.

73. Pontremoli R, Robaudo C, et al: Long-term minoxidil treatment in refractory hypertension and renal failure. Clin Nephrol 1991;35:39–43.

74. Saseen JJ, Carter BL, Brown TER, et al: Comparison of nifedipine alone or with diltiazem or verapamil in hypertension. Hypertension 1996;28:109–114.

75. Watkins J, Abbott EC, et al: Attenuation of hypotensive effect of propranolol and thiazide diuretics by indomethacin. BMJ 1960;281:702–705.

76. Dixey JJ, et al: The effects of naproxen and sulindac on renal function and their interaction with hydrochlorothiazide and piretanide in man. Br J Clin Pharmacol 1987; 23:55.

77. Wright JT Jr, et al: The effect of high-dose short-term ibuprofen on antihypertensive control with hydrochlorothiazide. Clin Pharmacol Ther 1989;46:440.

78. Klassen D, et al: Assessment of blood pressure during treatment with naproxen or ibuprofen in hypertensive patients treated with hydrochlorothiazide. J Clin Pharmacol 1993; 33:971.

79. Ebel DL, et al: Effect of sulindac, piroxicam, and placebo on the hypotensive effect of propranolol in patients with mild to moderate essential hypertension. Adv Ther 1985;2:31.

80. Radack KL, et al: Ibuprofen interferes with the efficacy of antihypertensive drugs. Ann Intern Med 1987;107:628.

81. Abate MA, et al: Interaction of indomethacin and sulindac with labetalol. Br J Clin Pharmacol 1991;31:363.

82. Johnson AG, Nguyen TV, Applstat M, Day RO: Do nonsteroidal anti-inflammatory drugs affect blood pressure? Ann Intern Med 1994;121:289–300.

83. Hawkins MM, Seelig CB: A case of acute renal failure induced by the coadministration of NSAIDs and captopril. N C Med J 1990;51:290.

84. Seelig CB, et al: Nephrotoxicity associated with concomitant ACE inhibitor and NSAID therapy. South Med J 1990;83:1144.

85. Morales JM, Rodriguez-Paternina E, Araque A, et al: Long-term effect of a calcium antagonist on renal function in hypertensive renal transplant patients on cyclosporine therapy: A 5-year prospective randomized study. Transplant Proc 1994;26:2598–2599.

86. Pegelow CH, Colangelo MS, et al: Natural history of blood pressure in sickle cell disease: Risks for stroke and death associated with relative hypertension in sickle cell anemia. Am J Med 1997;102:171–177.

87. Mathiesen ER, Homel E, et al: Efficacy of captopril in postponing nephropathy in normotensive insulin-dependent diabetes mellitus with microalbuminuria. BMJ 1991;303: 81–87.

88. Viberti G, Mogensen CE, et al: Effect of captopril on progression to clinical proteinuria in patients with insulin-dependent diabetes mellitus and microalbuminuria. JAMA 1994;271:275–279.
89. Ravid M, Savin H, et al: Long-term stabilizing effect of angiotensin converting enzyme inhibition on plasma creatinine and on proteinuria in normotensive type II diabetic patients. Ann Intern Med 1993;118:577–581.
90. Slataper R, Vicknair M, Sadler R, Bakris GL: ACE inhibition normalizes renal size and microalbuminuria in normotensive insulin dependent diabetic patients. J Diabetes Compl 1994;8:2–6.
91. Gaber L, Walton C, Brown S, Bakris GL: Effects of different antihypertensive treatments on morphologic progression of diabetic nephropathy in uninephrectomized dogs. Kidney Int 1994;46:161–169.
92. Parving HH, Anderson AR, et al: Early aggressive antihypertensive therapy reduces rate of decline in kidney function in diabetic nephropathy. lancet 1983;32:1175–1179.
93. Zeller K, Whittaker E, et al: Effect of restricting dietary protein on the progression of renal failure in patients with insulin-dependent diabetes mellitus. N Engl J Med 1991;324:78–84.
94. Bravo EL: Pheochromocytoma and mineralocorticoid hypertension. In Glassock RJ (ed): Current Therapy in Nephrology and Hypertension, 3rd ed. St. Louis, Mosby, 1992, pp 386–391.
95. Materson BJ, Reda DJ, Preston RA, et al: Response to a second single antihypertensive agent used as monotherapy for hypertension after failure of the initial drug. Arch Intern Med 1995;155:1757.
96. Villarosa IP, Bakris GL: Combination therapy for hypertension and renal disease in diabetes. In Mogensen CE (ed): The Kidney and Hypertension in Diabetes Mellitus, 4th ed. Boston, Kluwer Academic 1998, pp 569–579.

CHAPTER 5

Accelerated and Malignant Hypertension

I. **Definitions**
   A. **Malignant hypertension:** elevated diastolic blood pressure with at least one of the following
      1. Papilledema
      2. New central nervous system (CNS) alterations
         a. Especially abnormal mental status
         b. Differentiation from secondary hypertension due to stroke is sometimes difficult but critically important; funduscopic exam showing hemorrhages or exudates may help; hypertension due to stroke should be treated with extreme caution, if at all (see pages 17 and 70)
      3. New angina, myocardial infarct, or pulmonary edema
      4. Acute, progressive deterioration of renal function
   B. **Accelerated hypertension:** elevated diastolic blood pressure with at least one of the following
      1. Slowly rising creatinine
      2. Progressively rising blood pressures
      3. Worsening end-organ damage (e.g., congestive heart failure)

II. **Causes**
   A. **Preexisting hypertension:** patients are often 35–55 years old
   B. **Secondary hypertension**
      1. Birth control pills
      2. CNS disorder (e.g., cord tumors, Guillain-Barré syndrome)
      3. Acute glomerulonephritis
      4. Renovascular disorder
      5. Withdrawal of antihypertensive agents, especially beta blockers or clonidine
      6. Drug interactions (see Appendix VIII)
         a. Monoamine oxidase inhibitors
         b. Beta blockers with clonidine or methyldopa
         c. Beta blockers with sympathomimetics
      7. Vasculitis
      8. Preeclampsia (see also Chapter 6)
      9. Pheochromocytoma
      10. Sympathomimetics
         a. Cocaine
         b. Amphetamines
         c. High doses of others
      11. Scleroderma

III. **Evaluation**
   A. **History**
      1. Medications
         a. Over-the-counter medicines
         b. Illicit drugs (e.g., cocaine, amphetamines)
         c. Psychotropics
         d. Sympathomimetic inhalers and sprays
         e. Regular medications
      2. Medical history
         a. Renal disorders
         b. Cardiac disorders
            i. Congestive heart failure

      ii. Ischemic heart disease
    c. CNS disorder
  3. Review of systems
    a. Neurologic symptoms

      i. Headache   iii. Focality
      ii. Visual disturbances   iv. Nausea or vomiting

    b. Cardiac symptoms
      i. Chest pain
      ii. Dyspnea
    c. Severe abdominal, back, neck, or chest pain may suggest aneurysm
    d. Endocrine symptoms
      i. Paroxysms of dizziness, sweating, palpitations, headaches
      ii. Change in menstrual periods, hirsutism, amenorrhea

B. **Physical examination**
  1. Blood pressure
    a. Right and left arms
    b. Supine and standing
    c. One leg, if possible
    d. At least three readings taken several minutes apart
  2. Lungs
  3. Heart
  4. Extremities: pulse or perfusion asymmetry
  5. Neurologic status
  6. Fundi
  7. Neck
    a. Carotid arteries
    b. Tracheal tug may be due to aneurysm

C. **Laboratory tests**
  1. Electrolytes: hypokalemia is found in large percentage of patients with malignant hypertension and may not reflect autonomous hypermineralo-corticoidism
  2. Chemistry panel
  3. Urinalysis
  4. Electrocardiogram
  5. Chest radiograph
  6. Blood count
  7. Blood smear (schistocytes)
  8. Urine metanephrine/creatinine ratio
    a. Normal: < 1 μg/mg
    b. Many clinicians also do 24-hour urine measurements for meta-nephrine and catecholamines

IV. **Treatment**

A. **Establishment of treatment goal**
  1. In general, lower arterial pressure 20–25% over 4–6 hr to mean arterial pressure of about 135 or diastolic pressure of 100–110 mmHg
  2. Use lower pressures with aortic dissection
  3. Parenteral or rapid oral reduction of **asymptomatic "severe" high blood pressure** is not appropriate if patient meets no criteria for malignant hypertension.[1–5]

a. Risk may be considerable
b. Aggressive treatment based on pressure alone is common error
4. Generally in primary stroke, reduction of pressure is *not* currently recommended; when reduction seems desirable, much higher pressure goals (e.g., 120 mmHg diastolic) should be considered[6]

B. **Selection of specific agents**[7–9] (see also Appendix X)
  1. **Nitroprusside:** usually first choice
     a. Exceptions
        i. Aortic dissection—add beta blocker
        ii. Pregnancy—avoid if possible
     b. Monitor
        i. Thiocyanate levels (keep below 70–120 μg/ml [7–12 mg/dl] when used more than 2 days, especially in patients with renal impairment)
        ii. Anion gap, especially with liver impairment
           (a) Often first finding in cyanide toxicity
           (b) Cyanide levels do **not** correlate with thiocyanate levels
  2. **Preeclampsia** (parenteral) (see chapter 6)
     a. Hydralazine
     b. Labetalol
     c. Calcium channel blockers under study; may interact with magnesium sulfate to cause neuromuscular blockade and/or hypotension
     d. Minibolus diazoxide may be used
     e. Avoid angiotensin-converting enzyme (ACE) inhibitors
     f. Nitroprusside may cause cyanide toxicity, with potential harm to fetus, and should be reserved for hypertension unresponsive to other drugs in maximal doses
  3. **Sympathetic overactivity**
     a. Nitroprusside
     b. Phentolamine
     c. Labetalol (not alone in patients with pheochromocytoma; α:β = 1:7 ratio)
  4. **Maintenance**
     a. Start as soon as possible
     b. Consider calcium channel blockers, labetalol, and ACE inhibitors in patients without contraindications
     c. Many beta blockers may worsen renal blood flow
     d. Avoid early use of diuretics in absence of congestive heart failure or peripheral edema
  5. **Urgent hypertension** (see also Appendix X)
     a. Rapid lowering of pressure is not indicated in asymptomatic patients[2–5]
     b. Avoid large initial doses
     c. Avoid normalization of pressure
     d. Clonidine by mouth often safest[7]
     e. Use of sublingual or crushed oral nifedipine is no longer recommended for either severe asymptomatic hypertension or malignant hypertension
        i. Not absorbed sublingually
        ii. Drop in pressure may be profound and prolonged and has led to stroke and myocardial infarction

   iii. Nitroprusside is generally drug of choice for hypertensive emer-
    gencies because of its short half-life and rapid onset so that pro-
    longed hypotension can be avoided
   iv. Short-acting nifedipine has not been proved safe or effective for
    treatment of hypertension and is not approved by FDA for treat-
    ment of hypertension in any form
  6. In cocaine- or amphetamine-induced hypertension use extreme caution
   and short-acting drugs; for cocaine hypertension
   a. Drugs of choice: phentolamine, nitroglycerin, and verapamil[8]
   b. Nitroprusside has been used
   c. Avoid beta blockers because of increased risk of coronary ischemia[9]

V. **Drug Therapy**
 A. **Nitroprusside**
  1. Arteriolar and venous vasodilator
  2. No change in cardiac output
  3. **Starting dose:** 0.5 μg/kg/min
  4. **Maintenance:** increase dose by 0.5–1 μg/kg/min every 3 minutes
  5. Hepatic or renal insufficiency—increased toxicity if used more than 2–3
   days
   a. Keep thiocyanate below 100 μg/ml (10 mg/dl)
   b. Watch bicarbonate and anion gap (first abnormality in cyanide toxic-
    ity that is **not** reflected in thiocyanate levels)
   c. Antidotes
    i. Sodium nitrite
    ii. Sodium thiosulfate
    iii. Hydroxocobalamin
    iv. Hemodialysis (highly effective)
  6. In patients with **aortic dissection**, beta blocker **must** be used first
   a. 0.5 mg test dose of propranolol over 2 minutes
   b. Then 1 mg every 5 minutes to maximum of 0.15 mg/kg or heart rate
    of 60 bpm
   c. Maintenance: 2–6 mg every 4–6 hours
 B. **Diazoxide**
  1. Direct arteriolar vasodilator
  2. Reflex tachycardia and increase in cardiac output
  3. **Starting dose**
   a. No prior antihypertensives: 100-mg rapid bolus
   b. Prior antihypertensives: 50-mg rapid bolus
   c. Use smaller boluses in pregnancy (see Chapter 6)
  4. Peaks in 5 minutes
  5. Mainly used when constant monitoring is not possible and in pregnancy
   when pressure does not respond to other agents
 C. **Labetalol: initial dose**
  1. No prior drugs: 20 mg IV over 2 minutes
  2. Prior antihypertensives: 10 mg IV over 2 minutes
 D. **Nonparenteral regimens** (generally not recommended; see also Appendix X)
  1. Clonidine[7]
   a. Loading dose: 0.2 mg
   b. Further dose: 0.1 mg/hr until pressure improves or 0.7 mg total dose

2. Minoxidil and propranolol
   a. Starting dose: 10 mg of minoxidil and 40 mg of propranolol
   b. May repeat every 4 hours until goal reached and then go to mainte-
      nance schedule
   c. Eventually patient will need loop diuretic as well
   d. Adjust beta blocker to control tachycardia

VI. **Further Evaluation**

In addition to above, all patients who are suitable candidates should have reliable
evaluation for renal artery stenosis, such as magnetic resonance angiography
(MRA) or, preferably, intraarterial digital subtraction renal angiography

REFERENCES

1. Black HR, Cohan JD, et al: The Sixth Report of the Joint National Committee on
   Detection, Evaluation, and Treatment of High Blood Pressure (JNC VI). Arch Intern
   Med 1997;157:2413–2445.
2. Severe symptomless hypertension [editorial]. Lancet 1989;2:1369.
3. O'Mailia J, Sander GE, Giles TD: Nifedipine-associated myocardial ischemia or infarction
   in the treatment of hypertensive urgencies. Ann Intern Med 1987;107:185.
4. Zeller KR, Von Kuhnert L, Mathews C: Rapid reduction of severe asymptomatic hypertension: A prospective randomized trial. Arch Intern Med 1989;149:2186.
5. Fagan T: Acute reduction of blood pressure in asymptomatic patients with severe hypertension: An idea whose time has come—and gone [editorial]. Arch Intern Med 1989;149:
   2169–2170.
6. Powers WJ: Acute hypertension after stroke: The scientific basis for treatment decisions.
   Neurology 1993;43:461–467.
7. Anderson RJ, Hart GR, Crumpier CP, et al: Oral clonidine loading in hypertensive urgencies. JAMA 1981;246:848–850.
8. Pitts WR, Lange RA, et al: Cocaine-induced myocardial ischemia and infarction:
   Pathophysiology, recognition, and management. Prog Cardiovasc Dis 1997;40:65–76.
9. Bakris GL: Hypertension. In Stein JH (ed): Internal Medicine: Diagnosis and Therapy, 3rd
   ed. Norwalk, CN, Appleton & Lange, 1993, pp 171–187.

CHAPTER 6

Hypertension during Pregnancy

I. **Normal Pressure and Cardiac Function during Pregnancy**
   A. Diastolic blood pressure falls during first half of pregnancy
      1. Nadir: mid-second trimester
      2. Falls as much as 10 mmHg
      3. Normal diastolic pressure by end of second trimester: < 75 mmHg
   B. Pressure rises during second half of pregnancy
      1. By end of pregnancy, it is about equal to prepartum level
      2. Normal is defined as < 85 mmHg diastolic pressure in third trimester
      3. Regardless of initial pressure, **rise of 30 mmHg in systolic and/or 15 mmHg in diastolic pressure on two occasions represents hypertension in pregnancy**
      4. Diastolic pressure of 100 mmHg or greater is considered severe hypertension during pregnancy[1]
   C. Cardiac index increases by about 50% during first trimester and remains elevated thereafter

II. **Incidence of Hypertensive Problems during Pregnancy**
   A. 5–10% of all gestations
   B. 20% of all nulliparas
   C. 40–50% of all twinnings

III. **Classification and Features**
   A. **Preeclampsia–eclampsia**
      1. Causes 50% of hypertension of pregnancy
      2. Onset after 20th week
      3. More in nulliparas; much less in multiparas without prior episodes
      4. Prodrome (may occur with or without any of following)
         a. Headache—sign of severe disease   c. Hyperreflexia
         b. Severe epigastric pain—ominous   d. None of these may be present
      5. Features
         a. Hypertension
            i. May be mild
            ii. New onset in third trimester
         b. Edema alone is not abnormal in pregnancy
         c. Liver and coagulation abnormalities also may be present
         d. Uric acid elevation (> 4.4 mg/dl), in absence of diuretics, is earlier and more sensitive marker than proteinuria
         e. **Eclampsia**
            i. Defined as preeclampsia with seizures
            ii. Does not necessarily correlate with severity of features of preeclampsia; **all preeclamptics are at risk**
         f. **Hemolysis, elevated liver enzymes, and low platelet count (HELLP) syndrome**[4–7]
            i. Mild hypertension
            ii. Little proteinuria
            iii. Subtle hemolysis
            iv. Low platelet counts
            v. Abnormal liver function tests
            vi. Immediate indication of serious problem
            vii. Immediate termination of pregnancy is crucial
            viii. May become rapidly progressive condition

ix. **Differentiation from hemolytic-uremic syndrome (HUS) and thrombotic thrombocytopenic purpura (TTP) may be difficult** because of overlap of many manifestations (Table 13)

    (a) Almost all patients with HELLP syndrome show signs of resolution within 48–72 hr after termination of pregnancy

    (b) HELLP is much more common; HUS and TTP are **rare**

    (c) HELLP uncommonly has postpartum onset; TTP commonly begins postpartum

    (d) Fever and adenopathy are more common with HUS and TTP

    (e) Patients with HELLP often appear relatively healthy initially, with preceding laboratory abnormalities; patients with HUS and TTP usually appear critically ill from onset of illness

    (f) HELLP syndrome is treated with termination of pregnancy followed by supportive care; HUS and TTP usually are treated with plasma exchange

    (g) Antithrombin III is decreased in HELLP syndrome but not in HUS/TTP

g. Retinal arteriolar spasm (50% of patients)

h. Hyperreflexia

i. More common in

    i. Nulliparas

    ii. Older multiparas, especially if hypertensive

    iii. Patients living at higher altitudes

    iv. Patients with diabetes mellitus

    v. Patients with hydatidiform mole

    vi. Patients with preexisting hypertension with diastolic readings over 100 for 4 years previously[8]

    vii. Patients with chronic hypertension and prior episodes of preeclampsia[8]

B. **Chronic hypertension**

1. Most patients have underlying essential hypertension

2. Same differential diagnosis as ordinary hypertension

3. High incidence of superimposed preeclampsia

4. Generally slightly higher pressures are accepted

5. Drugs of choice for chronic hypertension in pregnancy[12]

    a. Methyldopa is first drug of choice

    b. Hydralazine may be added

    c. Beta-blockers may be used (may not be safe early in pregnancy, ***not to be used simultaneously with methyldopa***)

TABLE 13. Differential Diagnosis of HUS/TTP vs. HELLP

Findings	HUS/TTP	HELLP
Prevalence	Rare	Common
Usual presentation	Clinical illness	Asymptomatic with lab abnormalties
Postpartum presentation	Common	Rare
Fever	Common	Rare
Adenopathy	Common	Rare
Resolution	May not resolve spontaneously	Usually within 48–72 hr postpartum
Antithrombin III	Normal	Decreased

    d. Nifedipine may be added to above drugs with caution (limited data on safety for this indication)

    e. Low-dose diuretics started before pregnancy may be continued

        i. Avoid adding during pregnancy, as volume depletion may occur

    f. Avoid alpha blockers

    g. ACE inhibitors and angiotensin II receptor blockers are contraindicated

6. Goal is diastolic of 100 mmHg or less unless evidence of hypertension-induced symptoms or complications[12]

7. Chronic hypertensives with proteinuria ≥ 1 gm have worse fetal outcomes[8]

8. Patients generally do well except with secondary or complicated hypertension

    a. Polyarteritis and collagen vascular diseases have higher mortality rates

    b. Significantly azotemic patients do not do well without aggressive dialytic intervention

    c. Be sure to exclude **pheochromocytoma** with any suspicion

        i. Management of pheochromocytoma is pharmacologic until term in many patients, but tumors in dangerous locations, such as aortic bifurcation (organ of Zuckerkandl), may be increasingly troublesome as pregnancy progresses and are best removed early

        ii. Failure to diagnose before delivery may lead to death during or after delivery

        iii. Urinary and plasma catecholamines and metabolite tests are similar in pregnant and nonpregnant patients

        iv. Provocative testing is contraindicated

        v. Medical therapy: alpha blockers, as in nonpregnant patients

    d. **Hyperaldosteronism**

        i. Patients may become normokalemic during pregnancy[9]

        ii. Although aldosterone and renin levels may be elevated in normal pregnancy, suppression tests are valid

        iii. Spironolactone and angiotensin-converting enzyme (ACE) inhibitors are contraindicated during pregnancy

    e. **Cushing's syndrome:** critical to diagnose as early as possible

        i. 10% have malignant adrenal tumors

        ii. Diagnostic testing differs from nonpregnant patients

           (a) Overnight dexamethasone suppression tests show nonsuppression in normal pregnancy

           (b) Loss of diurnal variation is single most reliable screening test

           (c) High-dose suppression tests show suppression in normal pregnancy and in patients with adenomas

           (d) Adrenocorticotropic hormone (ACTH) levels are elevated in normal pregnancy

           (e) Ultrasound may detect adrenal mass

           (f) Localization is critical; MRI or CT of head and adrenal glands may be needed

        iii. Resection of tumor is critical and should not be delayed during pregnancy

C. **Chronic hypertension with superimposed preeclampsia**

    1. Poorest outcome

    2. High recurrence rate, even in multigravidas

D. **Late or transient hypertension**
1. Relatively benign condition with **no** manifestations except mild hypertension late in pregnancy
2. Precursor of essential hypertension[3]
3. Treat as preeclampsia if any question
4. Uric acid should be normal

E. **Late postpartum preeclampsia–eclampsia**
1. Days to 1–2 weeks after delivery
2. Rare

F. **Postpartum hypertension:** patient is normotensive during pregnancy and becomes hypertensive weeks later, eventually normalizing within 1 year

IV. **Pathophysiology in Preeclampsia**
A. Reversal of usual diurnal blood pressure variation: highest pressures at night
B. Labile pressure
C. Vascular hypersensitivity, particularly to angiotensin II (AII)
D. Decreased intravascular volume
E. Relatively decreased cardiac output
F. Low cardiac filling pressures
G. Fall in renal blood flow
H. Fall in glomerular filtration rate
I. Impairment of escape from hyperaldosteronism leads to sodium retention, edema, and hypertension
J. May be caused by imbalance in endogenous vasodilators and vasoconstrictors

V. **Management of Preeclampsia**
A. **Hospitalization** is strongly recommended
B. If patient normalizes in hospital, occasionally she may be followed at home, if trustworthy
C. Delivery at term: **never delay delivery at term**
D. **Worse prognosis** with any of following
1. Systolic pressure > 160 mmHg
2. Diastolic pressure > 110 mmHg
3. Protein excretion > 2 gm/24 hr or spot urine protein > 100 mg/dl
4. Increasing serum creatinine
5. Evidence of hemolysis, including schistocytes, high lactate dehydrogenase (LDH)
6. Epigastric or right upper abdominal pain
7. Severe headache or other central nervous system signs
8. Congestive heart failure
9. Retinal hemorrhages, exudates, or papilledema without other adverse prognostic findings suggests underlying preexistent chronic hypertension[3]
10. Intrauterine growth retardation

E. In patients who have not reached 34 weeks, attempt to stabilize may be made
1. If attempts to keep diastolic blood pressure below 105 mmHg (100 in teenagers) fail after 24–48 hours, delivery by cesarean section is mandatory
2. **Never** delay delivery if following signs or symptoms appear
   a. Worsening headache
   b. Worsening or severe epigastric pain
   c. Worsening or persistent hyperreflexia
   d. Failure to control blood pressure, as above

   e. Clotting abnormality, especially thrombocytopenia
   f. Liver function abnormalities
F. **Approach to treatment**
   1. Reduction of blood pressure to what level?
      a. Controversial
      b. Approximately 90–105 mmHg diastolic pressure
      c. Too low also may be harmful
   2. Bed rest: important to include some ambulation to avoid deep vein thrombosis[10]
   3. Treatment of choice in **all** patients past 34–36 weeks is immediate delivery
   4. If patient has **altered mentation, neurologic findings, altered liver function tests (2 times normal, especially with abdominal pain), low platelet count (< 100,000), pulmonary edema, 1-mg/dl rise in creatinine, persistent severe headache, or visual changes, deliver at any stage**
      a. Baby has better chance outside toxemic uterus
      b. Stable severe preeclamptics who are preterm may be referred to tertiary care center for expectant management in select cases[11,12] but otherwise should not be managed expectantly
   5. First drug of choice in absence of severe tachycardia is hydralazine: 5 mg IV, then 5–10 mg IV every 20–30 minutes (up to 20 mg)
   6. Many physicians use parenteral labetalol next
      a. 20-mg IV bolus every 10 minutes to maximum of 300 mg
      b. Follow bolus control with infusion, 1–2 mg/min (20–40 cc/hr of 800 mg/250 cc concentration)
   7. Miniboluses of diazoxide, 30 mg, also may be used
   8. Magnesium sulfate is used in most cases as adjunct and to prevent seizures
      a. Should be continued 24 hours postpartum (Table 14)
      b. May interact with calcium channel blockers to cause hypotension or neuromuscular blockade
   9. Although safe by some studies, beta blockers (other than labetalol) have not been well studied and may impair stress tolerance of fetus (see 15.e. on following page)
   10. Avoid all other medications
       a. Many are of unknown toxicity

TABLE 14. Use of Magnesium Sulfate ($MgSO_4$) in the Treatment of Preeclampsia

---

- 5–6 gm ($MgSO_4.7H_2O$) in 5% dextrose in water (D5W) IV piggyback over 20–30 minutes
- Then 1–2 gm/hr
- Keep levels between 6 and 9 mg/dl
- Increase dose for hyperreflexia
- Decrease dose for hyporeflexia, pending levels
- Additional 2–4 gm over 5–10 minutes after initial bolus if seizures persist
- 250 mg amobarbital IV over 3 minutes if seizures still persist
- Continue administration for 24 hours postpartum
- Keep an ampule of calcium gluconate at bedside for emergency treatment of hypermagnesemia

---

Modified from Wilton AG, Sibai BM: Hypertension in pregnancy: Current concepts of preeclampsia. Annu Rev Med 1997;48:115–127.

   b. Following drugs are **contraindicated**
      i. Nitroprusside (except when above options fail)
      ii. ACE inhibitors[13,14]
      iii. Ganglionic blockers
11. Although volume expansion was once advocated, it is no longer recommended because[15-18]
   a. Myocardial performance may be compromised
   b. Volume expansion with sodium may increase vascular reactivity
   c. Administration of nonprotein fluid decreases oncotic pressure, which may lead to pulmonary edema and cerebral edema
12. Volume expansion with colloid may be used when it seems mandatory, but only with monitoring of central pressures
13. Order liver ultrasound in any patient with persistent abdominal pain to rule out subcapsular hemorrhage (which may be fatal if untreated)
14. Diuretics are avoided except as last resort or with frank congestive heart failure; if fluid retention **due to medications** occurs, diuretics may be used **with caution**
15. **Chronic hypertension in absence of preeclampsia**
   a. 85% of patients do well
   b. More complications in patients over 30
   c. Methyldopa is still drug of choice in pregnancy for treatment of chronic hypertension
   d. Diuretics are generally avoided acutely but may be continued chronically if patient was salt-sensitive before pregnancy; discontinue if preeclampsia develops
   e. Use of beta blockers and labetalol may be associated with fetal growth retardation if used in early pregnancy.[19] Atenolol and some other beta blockers have adverse hemodynamic effects and should be avoided during pregnancy[20]
   f. ACE inhibitors and AII blockers are contraindicated during pregnancy
   g. Long-term outcome, risks, and benefits of calcium channel blockers have not been established, but if methyldopa and labetalol cannot be used or are ineffective, long-acting nifedipine may be considered if hypertension is severe[1]

VI. **Prevention**

Only low-dose aspirin has been shown (in small preliminary studies) to prevent preeclampsia. This treatment probably should be reserved for patients with prior preeclampsia and high risk of recurrence (e.g., patients with chronic essential hypertension over age 40 with history of preeclampsia)[21-24]

VII. **Follow-up**

   A. Evaluation at 3 months postpartum (in **all** patients)
      1. Blood pressure
      2. 24-hour urine protein
      3. Urine sediment
   B. All manifestations should have resolved by 3 months postpartum. Abnormal findings indicate underlying disease such as chronic glomerulonephritis. Such patients should be evaluated by nephrologist[2]

REFERENCES

1. Sibai BM: Treatment of hypertension in pregnant women. N Engl J Med 1996;335:257–265.
2. Brown MA, Whitworth JA: The kidney in hypertensive pregnancies—victim and villain. Am J Kidney Dis 1992;20:427–442.
3. Chua S, Redmond CWG: Prognosis for pre-eclampsia complicated by 5 g or more of proteinuria in 24 hours. Eur J Obstet Gynecol Reprod Biol 1992;43:9–12.
4. Pritchard JA, Weisman R, Ratnoff OD, Vosburgh GJ: Intravascular hemolysis, thrombocytopenia and other hematologic abnormalities associated with severe toxemia of pregnancy. N Engl J Med 1954;250:89–98.
5. Weinstein L: Syndrome of hemolysis, elevated liver enzymes, and low platelet count: A severe consequence of hypertension in pregnancy. Am J Obstet Gynecol 1982;142:159–167.
6. Killam AP, Dillard SH, Patton RC, Pederson PR: Pregnancy-induced hypertension complicated by acute liver disease and disseminated intravascular coagulation: Five case reports. Am J Obstet Gynecol 1975;123:823–828.
7. Miller JM, Pastorek JG: Thrombotic thrombocytopenic purpura and hemolytic uremic syndrome in pregnancy. Clin Obstet Gynecol 1991;34:64–71.
8. Sibai BM, Lindheimer M, Hauth J, et al: Risk factors for preeclampsia, abruptio placentae, and adverse neonatal outcomes among women with chronic hypertension. N Engl J Med 1998;339:667–671.
9. August P, Sealey JE: The renin-angiotensin system in normal and hypertensive pregnancy and ovarian function. In Laragh JH, Brenner BM (eds): Hypertension: Pathophysiology, Diagnosis and Management. New York, Raven Press, 1990, pp 1761–1768.
10. Brown MA: Nonpharmacological management of pregnancy induced hypertension. J Hypertens 1990;8:295–301.
11. Wilton AG, Sibai BM: Hypertension in pregnancy: Current concepts of preeclampsia. Annu Rev Med 1997;115–127.
12. August P, Rose BD: Hypertension and Proteinuria in Pregnancy. Up To Date 1998;6(3) (CD ROM).
13. Smith AM: Are ACE inhibitors safe in pregnancy? [editorial]. Lancet 1989;2:750–751.
14. Hennessey A, Horvath JS: Newer antihypertensive agents in pregnancy. Med J Aust 1992;156:304–305.
15. Sibai BM, et al: Pulmonary edema in severe preeclampsia–eclampsia: Analysis of thirty seven consecutive cases. Am J Obstet Gynecol 1984;156:1174–1179.
16. Benedetti TJ, Kates R, Williams V: Hemodynamic observations in severe preeclampsia complicated by pulmonary edema. Am J Obstet Gynecol 1985;152:330–334.
17. Benedetti TJ, Quilligan EJ: Cerebral edema in severe pregnancy-induced hypertension. Am J Obstet Gynecol 1980;137:860–862.
18. Pritchard JA, Cunningham FG, Pritchard SA: The Parkland Memorial Hospital protocol for treatment of eclampsia: Evaluation of 245 cases. Am J Obstet Gynecol 1984;148:951–963.
19. Sturgis SN, Lindheimer MD, Davison JM: Treatment of hypertension during pregnancy: Drugs to be avoided and drugs to be used. In Andreucci VE, Fine LG (eds): International Yearbook of Nephrology. New York, Springer-Verlag, 1991, pp 163–196.
20. Butters L, Kennedy S, Rubin PC: Atenolol in essential hypertension during pregnancy. BMJ 1990;301:587–589.
21. Beaufuls M, uzan S, Donsimoni R, Colau JC: Prevention of preeclampsia by early antiplatelet therapy. Lancet 1985;1:840–842.
22. Wallenberg HCS, Dekker GA, Makovitz JW, Rotmans P: Low dose aspirin prevents pregnancy-induced hypertension and preeclampsia in angiotensin-sensitive primigravidae. Lancet 1986;1:1–3.
23. Benigni A, Gregorini G, Frusca T, et al: Effect of low-dose aspirin on fetal and maternal generation of thromboxane by platelets in women at risk for pregnancy induced hypertension. N Engl J Med 1989;321:357–362.
24. Schiff E, Peleg E, Goldenberg M, et al: The use of aspirin to prevent pregnancy induced hypertension and lower the ratio of thromboxane A2 to prostacyclin in relatively high risk pregnancies. N Engl J Med 1986;321:351–356.

Approach to the Patient with Suspected Cushing's Syndrome

APPENDIX I

Approach to the Patient with Suspected Cushing's Syndrome

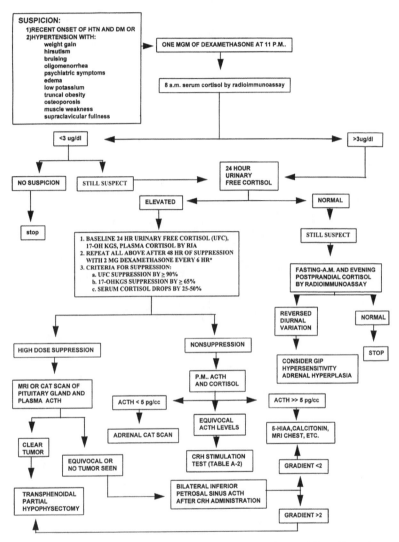

* A high-dose overnight test uses a single 8-mg dose of dexamethasone followed by a plasma cortisol the following morning; this test is an alternative (though not as established).

The patient suspected of having Cushing's syndrome will have some or all of the characteristics listed at the top of the chart. A simple screening test is the overnight dexamethasone suppression test. False positives occur with varying frequency (Table A1). To improve reliability, **use only radioimmunoassay measurements of cortisol**. With high suspicion, however, this test should not be relied on to rule out the diagnosis absolutely. A 24-hour urinary free cortisol test is usually diagnostic.

TABLE A1. False Results in the Overnight Dexamethasone Suppression Test and Urinary Free Cortisol Test

Overnight Dexamethasone Suppression Test		Urinary Free Cortisol Test
False positives	**False negatives**	**False positives**
Common	Ketoconazole	Uncommon
Acute psychiatric stress		Diuretics
Depression		High sodium diet
Uncommon		
Diphenylhydantoin (phenytoin)		
Alcohol		
Rifampin		
Birth control pills		

If the patient has a normal urinary cortisol, in the face of convincing clinical findings suggestive of Cushing's syndrome, a check of the plasma cortisol for reversal of the normal diurnal variation may be useful. An afternoon value higher than the fasting value is suggestive of the syndrome of gastric inhibitory peptide (GIP) hypersensitivity.[1,2] If urinary free cortisol is elevated, 24-hour urinary free cortisol 17-hydroxycorticosteroids (17-OHKGS = 17-hydroxyketogenic steroids), and plasma cortisol are measured before and after high-dose dexamethasone suppression (given as 2 mg every 6 hours). If urinary free cortisol is suppressed ≥ 90% along with suppression of 17-hydroxysteroids ≥ 65%, pituitary Cushing's syndrome is strongly suspected.

An overnight high-dose dexamethasone suppression test has recently been described and seems reliable. The only difficulties with this test are the relatively small number of patients studied and the fact that the test has been validated only in hospitalized patients.[3–5]

Nonsuppression leads to measurement of adrenocorticotropic hormone (ACTH) and search for ectopic secretion of ACTH. Such tests include hydroxyindoleacetic acid (5-HIAA) for carcinoid tumors and magnetic resonance imaging (MRI) of the chest and/or other appropriate locations. Computed tomography (CT) scanning and MRI are probably equivalent for pituitary imaging in the case of high-dose suppression. Failure to see a clear tumor justifies sampling of bilateral inferior petrosal sinus ACTH levels after administration of corticotropin-releasing factor (CRF). Lack of a difference between the two sides leads to further search for the unusual ectopic ACTH source that is suppressible. For workup during pregnancy see page 76.

TABLE A2. The CRH Stimulation Test[5]

Protocol
1. Obtain baseline ACTH and cortisol levels.
2. Administer 1 μg/kg or 100 μg of CRH at about 8:00 AM.
3. Obtain blood samples for ACTH and cortisol at 15-minute intervals for at least 2 hours.
4. Test valid only in untreated state.

Interpretation
1. Normal: flat or slightly rising curve; normal baseline ACTH.
2. Pituitary: sharp rise in ACTH (even to fivefold or more) with concomitant rise in cortisol; usually elevated baseline ACTH.
3. Adrenal: relatively flat curve; suppressed baseline ACTH.
4. Ectopic ACTH: relatively flat curve; higher baseline ACTH.

REFERENCES

1. Reznick YR, Veronique A, Chayvialle JA, et al: Food dependent Cushing's syndrome mediated by aberrant adrenal sensitivity to gastric inhibitory polypeptide. N Engl J Med 1992; 327:981–986.
2. Lacroix A, Bolte E, Tremblay J, et al: Gastric inhibitory polypeptide-dependent cortisol hypersecretion—a new cause of Cushing's syndrome. N Engl J Med 1992;327:974–980.
3. Tyrell JB, Findling JW, et al: An overnight high-dose dexamethasone suppression test for rapid differential diagnosis of Cushing's syndrome. Ann Intern Med 1986;104:180–186.
4. Bruno OD, Rossi MA, et al: Nocturnal high-dose dexamethasone suppression test in the aetiological diagnosis of Cushing's syndrome. Acta Endocrinol (Copenh) 1985;109:158–162.
5. Kaye TB, Crapo L: The Cushing syndrome: An update on diagnostic tests. Ann Intern Med 1990;112: 434–444.
6. Findling JW, Mazzaferri EL: Cushing syndrome—an etiologic workup. Hosp Pract 1992; 27:107–122.
7. Orth DN: Cushing's syndrome. N Engl J Med 1995;332:791–803.

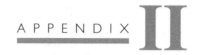

Approach to the Patient with Suspected Hyperaldosteronism

APPENDIX II

Approach to the Patient with Suspected Hyperaldosteronism

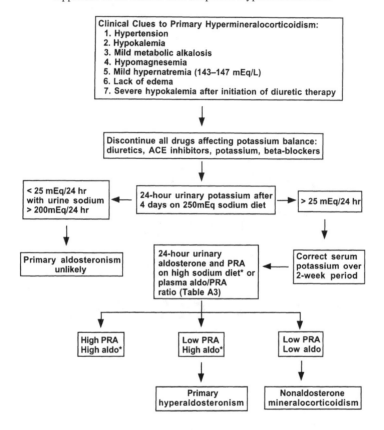

FIGURE A2.   Initial evaluation of patients with suspected hypermineralocorticoidism. The evaluation of the patient with suspected hypermineralocorticoidism starts with clinical suspicion, which may include any or all of the factors listed. Mild hypokalemia in a patient taking diuretics is not by itself grounds for further evaluation. On the other hand, some patients with various forms of hypermineralocorticoidism may be normokalemic, especially on a sodium-restricted diet. Most patients with correctable disease, however, are believed to be hypokalemic.

Evaluation starts with a 24-hour urinary potassium and sodium determination. Low urinary potassium (< 25–30 mEq/24 hr) in the presence of adequate salt intake (> 200 mEq/day off diuretics) excludes hypermineralocorticoidism. If urinary potassium is elevated, the next step is to evaluate the renin-aldosterone axis after potassium repletion (potassium is a major regulator of aldosterone secretion). In many cases of primary hyperaldosteronism, aldosterone (ALDO) is unsuppressed and renin suppressed; however, in some patients with proven primary hyperaldosteronism renin activity may not suppress (*see Fig. A3). Patients with inappropriate kaliuresis while on a high-salt diet and suppressed aldosterone should be investigated for alternative mineralocorticoids if no other explanation is apparent (such as estrogen administration, renovascular disease, malignant hypertension, or salt-wasting nephropathy; see Fig. A5 and Table A8). Aldosterone secretion is suppressed by hypokalemia, and this effect overcomes the effects of distal sodium delivery on potassium excretion in normal people.[2,3] Patients with high plasma renin activity and high aldosterone may have renal artery stenosis or, rarely, a renin-secreting tumor of the kidney (perihemangiocytoma) or ectopic secretion of renin from another tumor (e.g., oat cell carcinoma of the lung).

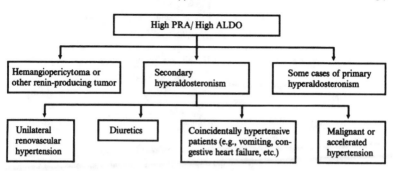

FIGURE A3. Differential diagnosis of hypokalemic hypertensive patients with high plasma renin activity and high aldosterone levels.

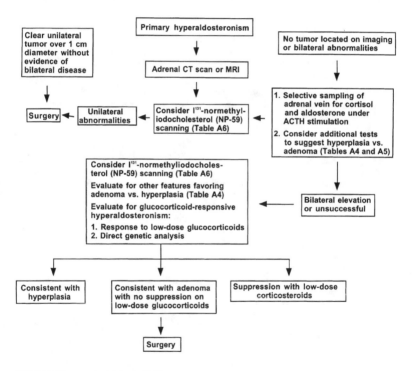

* These tests are not widely available.

FIGURE A4. Approach to the patient with confirmed hyperaldosteronism. The evaluation of a patient with confirmed hyperaldosteronism requires further testing to determine if the cause is primary adrenal hyperplasia, a solitary adenoma, or glucocorticoid-suppressible hyperaldosteronism (GSHA). Because GSHA is uncommon, even small adrenal tumors must be excluded first (with adrenal vein aldosterone, if necessary). When adrenal venous sampling is done, high ACTH-stimulated cortisol relative to mixed blood, in each adrenal vein specimen, assures the physician that the specimen was indeed obtained from the adrenal vein. Because bilateral abnormalities on MRI or CT may not represent functional adrenal hyperplasia, the diagnosis in such circumstances should be confirmed with additional tests such as those in Tables A4, A5, and/or an I^{131}-iodocholesterol scan (Table A6).

TABLE A3. Plasma Aldosterone/Renin Activity Screening Test for Primary Hyperaldosteronism

1. Patient must be normokalemic.
2. Patient must not be taking diuretics, ACE inhibitors, or high-dose beta blockers.
3. Criteria for positive test:
   a. PA (ng/dl)/PRA (ng/ml/hr) > 30
      and
   b. PA > 20 ng/dl
4. Acute administration of captopril 60–90 minutes before the test may increase sensitivity.

PA = plasma aldosterone; PRA = plasma renin activity.

TABLE A4. Tests in the Differentiation of Adrenal Hyperplasia vs. Solitary Adrenal Adenoma*

Test	Unilateral	Bilateral
Plasma aldosterone change with upright posture (Table A5)	Increased ≥ 33%	Decreased or unchanged
Ratio of 18-hydroxycorticosterone to cortisol after normal saline infusion over 2 hr (most useful test)	< 3	> 3
Urinary hydroxycortisol[†] and/or oxocortisol[†]	Low	High
Urinary aldosterone response to spironolactone	Increased	Decreased

* Some authors, most notably Biglieri,[3] suggest that patients with the findings characteristic of unilateral adenomas, who have histologic hyperplasia, also may respond to unilateral adrenalectomy.
[†] These tests not widely available.

TABLE A5. Protocol for Determination of Postural Variation in Plasma Aldosterone

Protocol
1. Discontinue spironolactone and ACE inhibitors for several weeks before study.
2. Place patient on 150 mEq (3.5-gm)/d sodium diet for 5 days.
3. Place patient in lying position overnight.
4. At 7 AM, with patient remaining supine, place indwelling catheter for blood drawing.
5. Draw 8 AM plasma aldosterone, 18-hydroxycorticosterone, potassium, cortisol, and PRA.
6. Repeat same tests upright at noon after 4 hours of ambulation.

Interpretation
1. Normal patients have a 2- to 4-fold rise in aldosterone.
2. Most patients with hyperplasia and some with unilateral adenomas have at least a 33% rise in aldosterone.
3. About half of patients with unilateral adenoma have little or no change.
4. The test is invalid if the cortisol level fails to drop with the noon measurement.

TABLE A6. I[131]-Methylnoriodocholesterol (NP59) Scanning

1. Give dexamethasone 1 mg by mouth 4 times/day starting 1 week before isotope injection; continue for a total of 10 days to suppress normal adrenal tissue.
2. Starting 2 days before isotope injection, give 1 drop SSKI by mouth 3 times/day; continue for 2 weeks (to protect thyroid).
3. Inject 5 mCi of ^{131}I-iodomethyl-19-norcholesterol (NP59) 1 week after initiation of dexamethasone and 3 days after initiation of SSKI.
4. Intercurrent [99m]Te-DTPA or glucoheptonate scans may be used for anatomic reference.
5. Some authors recommend a routine radiologic bowel preparation.
6. Interpretation of results:
   a. Bilateral uptake usually seen in hyperplasia.
   b. Unilateral hot area usually seen with adenoma.
   c. Carcinoma often cold bilaterally.

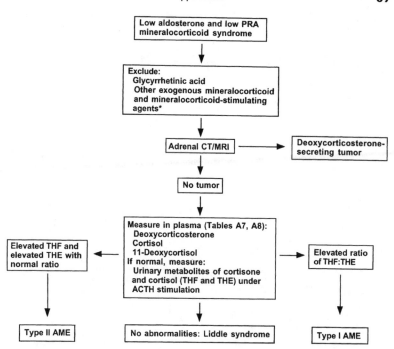

FIGURE A5.   **Evaluation of the patient with suspected hyperaldosteronism and low renin and aldosterone.** *Mineralocorticoid-stimulating or mineralocorticoid-like agents include carbenoxolone, fluorinated steroids, licorice and licorice-flavored tobacco, laxatives, and beverages. AME = apparent mineralocorticoid excess syndrome.

TABLE A7.   Summary of Test Results in Hypermineralocorticoid States

Entity	[K]	PRA	ALDO	ACTH	17-KS	RVR	DOC
Primary hyper-aldosteronism	L/N	L	H	N	N	N	L
Glucocorticoid responsive hyper-aldosteronism	N/L	L	H	H/N	N	N	L
Cushing's syndrome	N/L	N/H	N/H	L/H	N/H	N	N/H
Liddle syndrome	L	L	L	N	N	N	N
11-OH deficiency	N/L	L	L	N/H	H	—	H
17-OH deficiency	L	L	L	N/H	L	—	H
DOC tumor	L	L	L	L/N	N	—	H
Licorice or apparent mineralocorticoid excess	L	L	L	N	N	N	N
Hemangiopericytoma and ectopic renin	L	H	H	N	N	N/H	H
Renovascular hyper-tension	N/L	N/H	N/H	N	N	N/H	N

[K] = serum potassium; PRA = plasma renin activity; ALDO = aldosterone; DOC = deoxy-corticosterone; ACTH = adrenocorticotropic hormone; 17-KS = 17-ketosteroid; RVR = renal vein renin; 11-OH = 11-hydroxylase; 17-OH = 17-hydroxylase; L = low; N = normal; H = high.

TABLE A8. Tests in the Differential Diagnosis of Non-aldosterone Mineralocorticoidism

Entity	Plasma Metabolites			Urine Metabolites		
	F	DOC	11-Deoxy F	THF	THE	THF:THE
Licorice	N	N	N	H	L	>>1
Apparent mineralocorticoid excess type I *or* 11-beta hydroxysteroid dehydrogenase deficiency	N	N	N	H	L	>>1
Apparent mineralocorticoid excess type II	N/H	N	N	H	H	N
11-Beta hydroxylase deficiency	L	H	H	L	L	N
17-Hydroxylase deficiency	L	H	L	L	L	N
Liddle syndrome	N	N	N	N	N	N
Cortisol resistance	H	H	H	H	H	N

F = cortisol; DOC = doxycorticosterone; THF = tetrahydrocortisol; THE = tetrahydrocortisone; THF:THE = ratio of THF to THE (normally about 1.0).

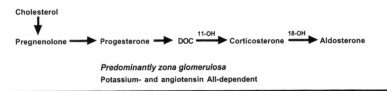

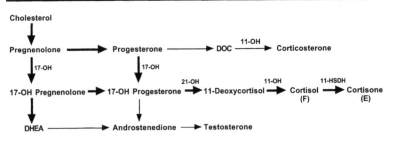

Predominantly zona fasciculata and reticularis
ACTH-dependent, cortisol is only feedback mechanism

FIGURE A6. **Metabolic pathways and defects in hypermineralocorticoid states.** Heavy arrows indicate normal major pathways; light arrows indicate minor pathways that may become important in certain disease states.

1. ACTH stimulation of the adrenal cortex results in increased production of cortisol, which, in turn, feeds back to suppress secretion of ACTH.

2. Angiotensin II stimulates the secretion of aldosterone.

3. Failure of cortisol production for any reason leads to increased ACTH release and therefore increased synthesis of steroids to the points in the metabolic pathways where the involved enzyme is deficient or inhibited.

4. Because 21-hydroxylase (21-OH) deficiency blocks the pathway to all mineralocorticoids, patients with this disorder have a tendency toward hyperkalemia and are normotensive or even salt-wasting. Androgens also accumulate.

5. In 11-hydroxylase (11-OH) deficiency, deoxycorticosterone (DOC), a potent mineralo-corticoid, and 11-deoxycortisol accumulate, as do the androgens.

6. In 17-hydroxylase deficiency, not only does deoxycorticosterone accumulate, but the pathway to sex steroids is blocked, as is the pathway to cortisol.

7. Normally aldosterone is produced only in the zona glomerulosa and not in the zona fas-ciculata, where ACTH acts preferentially. Aldosterone synthase is part of the aldosterone synthase complex which also contains 11-hydroxylase and 18-hydroxylase (CYP11B2). Aldosterone synthase is normally limited to the zona glomerulosa. In glucocorticoid-respon-sive hyperaldosteronism, it is also present in the zona fasciculata; this results in ordinary ACTH promoting the synthesis of aldosterone. This disorder is treated with ACTH suppres-sion via exogenous glucocorticoid. DHEA = dihydroxyepiandrosterone; 18-OH = 18-hydrox-ylase; 11-HSDH = 11-hydroxysteroid dehydrogenase.

REFERENCES

1. Biglieri EG: Spectrum of mineralocorticoid hypertension. Hypertension 1991;17:251–261.
2. Rose BD: Clinical Physiology of Acid-Base and Electrolyte Disorders, 3rd ed. New York, McGraw-Hill, 1993, pp 722–730.
3. Bravo EL, Tarazi RC, Dustan H, et al: The changing clinical spectrum of primary hyperal-dosteronism. Am J Med 1983;74:641–651.
4. Bakris GL, Mazzaferri EL: Severe hypertension in a young patient. Hosp Pract 1993;28: 57–64.
5. Slataper RM, Bakris GL: Secondary hypertension. In Taylor R (ed): Difficult Diagnosis II. Philadelphia, W.B. Saunders, 1992, pp 403–411.
6. Young WF, Hogan MJ, Klee GG, et al: Primary aldosteronism: Diagnosis and treatment. Mayo Clin Proc 1990;65:96–110.

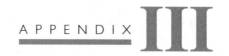
Workup and Management of Pheochromocytoma

APPENDIX III

Workup and Management of Pheochromocytoma

I. **Approach to Diagnosis of a Pheochromocytoma (Fig. A7)**[1,2]

A. In patients in whom the diagnosis is suspected, 24-hour urinary normetanephrine assay is the most reliable single test; total metanephrine is also a consistently good test.[3] Vanillylmandelic acid (VMA) and urinary catecholamines are less sensitive and have both lower sensitivity and and low specificity; however, measurements of **free (not total)** urinary catecholamines and VMA by **fluorometric assay after high-pressure liquid chromatography** (HPLC) separation have much greater reliability than older (but still commonly used) methods.[1] It is important to know which assays are used with HPLC methods.[1] Table A9 lists tests with high reliability.

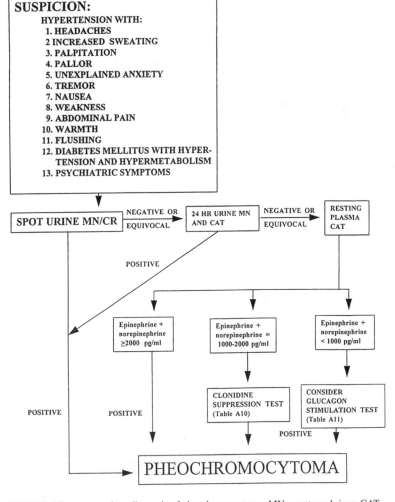

FIGURE A7. Approach to diagnosis of pheochromocytoma. MN = metanephrines; CAT = catecholamines; CR = creatinine.

TABLE A9. Interpretation of 24-hour Urinary Results in Patients with Suspected Pheochromocytoma

Test	Normal Values	Usual Values in Pheochromocytoma	Interference
Normetanephrine (fluorometric)	≤ 0.720 mg/24 hr	> 2 mg/24 hr Values < 0.720 mg/24 hr are rare	MAOIs Beta blockers Exogenous cate-cholamines Tetracyclines Acetaminophen
Total metanephrines	≤ 1.3 mg/24 hr	> 2 mg/24 hr	Same
Vanillylmandelic acid (VMA) (best after HPLC)	≤ 7 mg/24 hr	> 14 mg/24 hr	Carbidopa Methyldopa Clofibrate Disulfiram MAOIs Sinemet Reserpine Nitroglycerin Exogenous cate-cholamines
Urinary free (not conjugated) catecholamines (E + NE) (best after HPLC)	< 150 µg/24 hr	≥ 240 µg/24 hr	Methyldopa Ganglionic blockers Radiographic dye Reserpine Catecholamines Acetaminophen Alcohol L-dopa Methenamine Mandelamine Nicotine Nitroglycerin Erythromycin Tetracyclines Theophylline B vitamins in large doses Beta blockers Bananas

MAOIs = monoamine oxidase inhibitors; E = epinephrine; NE = norepinephrine; HPLC = high-pressure liquid chromatography.

TABLE A10. Clonidine Suppression Test[4-6]

Procedure[4,5]

1. Discontinue antihypertensives 12 hours before test.
2. Be sure that patient is volume-repleted.
3. Place heparin lock for blood drawing 30 minutes before drawing blood.
4. Thirty minutes after heparin lock is inserted, draw baseline plasma catecholamines (PC); put blood on ice.
5. Administer 0.3 mg of clonidine by mouth.
6. Redraw three more PC specimens at 1-hr intervals over the next 3 hours.

Interpretation

1. Normal suppression by 50% to < 500 pg/ml.
2. Results are invalid without elevated resting level.[6]
3. Volume repletion before test is mandatory, or profound hypotension may result.

TABLE AII.   Glucagon Stimulation Test for Patients Suspected of Having
Pheochromocytoma But with Catecholamines Below 1000 pg/ml

Procedure[2,3,7,8]
1. Pretreat patient with alpha blocker or calcium channel blocker.
2. Place heparin lock for blood drawing 30 minutes before test.
3. Draw baseline plasma catecholamines.
4. Give 1 mg of intravenous glucagon.

Interpretation
Patients with pheochromocytoma have 3-fold or greater increase in catecholamines or absolute value > 2000 pg/ml.

    B. During **paroxysms** patients may be asked to empty their bladder for double-voided spot **urinary metanephrine/creatinine ratio**
1. Test urine metanephrine/creatinine while patient is hypertensive
2. Values over 1 μg/mg (metanephrine/creatinine) are abnormal
3. Particularly useful as double-voided specimen after rise in pressure
4. Should be confirmed with fractionated urinary 24-hour tests

    C. Plasma catecholamines are useful in confirming the diagnosis, especially in equivocal cases
1. Procedure: resting, supine, heparin lock in place 1 hour before test
2. Diagnostic
    a. Norepinephrine > 2000 pg/ml (12 nmol/L)
    b. Epinephrine > 200 pg/ml (1.1 nmol/L)
3. Nondiagnostic elevations may be caused by
    a. Anxiety
    b. Smoking
    c. Exercise
    d. Pheochromocytoma
4. Potentially useful in borderline cases, especially with clonidine suppression, which does not suppress result in pheochromocytoma

II. **Localization of Pheochromocytomas (Fig. A8)**
    A. Because 5% of pheochromocytomas occur in setting of multiple endocrine neoplasia syndrome type II (MEN II), beware of possibility of medullary carcinoma of thyroid as well as hyperparathyroidism
    B. Computed tomography is positive in 90% of cases
    C. Because bladder tumors are common site of extraadrenal tumors, intravenous pyelogram with views of bladder may be valuable if CT scanning is not diagnostic
    D. ^{131}I-metaiodobenzylguanidine (MIBG) scans (Table A12) pick up most of the rest but are not widely available
    E. Scanning of mediastinum and, rarely, elsewhere may be needed.
    F. Occasionally adrenal venographic sampling is still necessary

III. **Preoperative Management of Pheochromocytoma**
    A. First a long-acting alpha blocker (phenoxybenzamine) is used for maximal inhibition of postsynaptic alpha receptors (as evidenced by ≥ 20 mmHg drop in blood pressure after standing)
    B. Calcium channel blockers can then be added; beta blockade occasionally may be needed in patients with high epinephrine-like activity **but only after maximal alpha blockade**
    C. Volume expansion preoperatively is **critical**

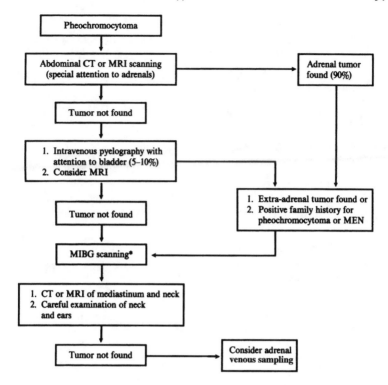

FIGURE A8. Approach to localization of pheochromocytoma. * Available only at very few centers.

1. Such patients have greatest need for volume expansion compared with other causes of secondary hypertension
2. Give at least 2–5 L of normal saline
3. Administer under hemodynamic monitoring if necessary
D. **Beware of factitious exogenous catecholamine administration** in strange cases, especially among health care professionals

TABLE A12.　[131]I-Metaiodobenzylguanidine (MIBG) Scanning for Localization of Pheochromocytoma

1. Screen for factors that may interfere with test (Table A13) and substitute for interfering drugs at least 24 hr in advance.
2. Give 100 mg of iodide as Lugol's solution or SSKI at time of isotope administration.
3. Administer 7–14 μCi/kg of ^{131}I-MIBG.
4. Do scan 24 hours after ^{131}I-MIBG; include skull through pelvis.

TABLE A13.　Substances that May Interfere with MIBG Scanning

Reserpine	Tricyclic antidepressants	? Chocolate
Phenothiazines	Pseudoephedrine, phenylpropanolamine,	? Vanilla
Labetalol	other sympathomimetic amines	? Clonidine
Cocaine	Amphetamines	? Certain cheeses

REFERENCES

1. Stein PP, Black HR: A simplified diagnostic approach to pheochromocytoma. A review of the literature and report of one institution's experience. Medicine 1990;70:46–66.

2. DeQuattro V, Meyers M, Campese VM: Pheochromocytoma: Diagnosis and therapy. In Degroot LJ, Besser GM, Cahill GF, et al (eds): Endocrinology. Philadelphia, W.B. Saunders, 1989, pp 1780–1797.

3. Manu P, Runge LA: Biochemical screening for pheochromocytoma: Superiority of urinary metanephrines measurements. Am J Epidemiol 1984;120:788–790.

4. Bravo EL, Terazi RC, Fouad F, et al: Clonidine suppression test: A useful aid in the diagnosis of pheochromocytoma. N Engl J Med 1981;305:623–626.

5. Grossman E, Goldstein DS, Hoffman A, Keiser HR: Glucagon and clonidine testing in the diagnosis of pheochromocytoma. Hypertension 1991;17:733–741.

6. Elliot WJ, Murphy MB: Reduced specificity of the clonidine suppression test in patients with normal plasma catecholamine levels. Am J Med 1988;84:419–424.

7. Sheps SG, Jiang N, Klee GG, et al: Recent developments in the diagnosis and treatment of pheochromocytoma. Mayo Clin Proc 1990;65:88–95.

8. Bravo EM: Pheochromocytoma: New concepts and future trends. Kidney Int 1991;40: 544–556.

9. Setaro JF, Black HR: Current concepts: Refractory hypertension. N Engl J Med 1992; 327:543–547.

10. Yi J, Bakris GL: Pheochromocytoma. In Conn RB, Borer WZ, Snyder JW (eds): Current Diagnosis, 9th ed. Philadelphia, W.B. Saunders, 1997, pp 794–798.

Approach to the Patient with Suspected Renovascular Hypertension

APPENDIX IV

Approach to the Patient with Suspected Renovascular Hypertension[1-5]

When deciding which path to follow in investigating a patient who may have renovascular hypertension, the clinician is faced with several questions. If the patient is not a candidate for angioplasty or surgery, there is little point in pursuing the diagnosis. If the patient has average risk and the clinician is strongly suspicious, direct intraarterial digital subtraction angiography has been the standard approach with the highest sensitivity and specificity. Many patients fall outside these two groups and may be at risk from angiography, contrast dye, or both, and yet there may be some suspicion. In these cases, the safest procedure may be the captopril isotope renogram. More recently, the spiral CT scan of the renal arteries has been introduced. It has high sensitivity and high specificity but has the disadvantage of requiring use of intravenous contrast material. On the other hand, it may provide anatomical information that the isotopic study may not.[6,7] Specialized "3-D time of flight" magnetic resonance angiography[8,9] has become available in the last few years. It offers the advantage of anatomical information without the high risk associated with contrast material. Its contraindications include aneurysm clips, pacemakers, and other circumstances. It also offers high sensitivity and specificity. Most recently, very high-quality detailed images have been obtained using gadolinium-enhanced magnetic resonance angiography (GE-MRA). This procedure provides information that

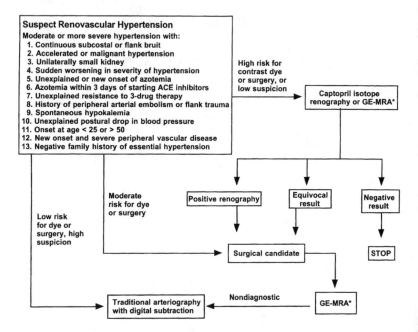

*GE-MRA = gadolinium-enhanced "fast" magnetic resonance angiography.

FIGURE A9. Evaluation of the patient with suspected renovascular hypertension.
Protocol for captopril isotope renography is shown in Table A14.

TABLE A14.   Protocol for Captopril Isotopic Renography

1. Stop ACE inhibitors 24 hours before test; stop diuretics 1 week before test if possible; check urine sodium to confirm that patient is sodium-replete.

2. Give 24 ounces of water 1 hour before test.

3. Check blood pressure.

4. Give 50 mg of crushed captopril by mouth.*

5. One hour later do DTPA renography.

DTPA = ^{99m}Tc-diethylenetriaminepentaacetate.

* Because of severe postural hypotension after captopril administration in some patients, it may become necessary to administer intravenous saline.

is superior to previous MRA studies and is nearly equal to formal conventional intraarterial angiography. It may be less useful in cases of vasculitis and small-vessel fibromuscular dysplasia.[10]

REFERENCES

1. Slataper RM, Bakris GL: Secondary hypertension. In Taylor R (ed): Difficult Diagnosis II. Philadelphia, W.B. Saunders, 1992, pp 403–411.

2. Rudnick MR, Maxwell MH: Limitations of renin assays. In Narins RS (ed): Controversies in Nephrology and Hypertension. New York, Churchill Livingstone, 1984, pp 123–160.

3. McCarthy JE, Weder AB: The captopril test and renovascular hypertension: A cautionary tale. Arch Intern Med 1990;150:493–495.

4. Setaro JF, Saddler MC, Chen CC, et al: Simplified captopril renography in the diagnosis and treatment of renal artery stenosis. Hypertension 1991;18:289–298.

5. Davidson R, Wilcox CS: Diagnostic usefulness of renal scanning after angiotensin converting enzyme inhibitors [editorial]. Hypertension 1991;18:299–303.

6. Olbricht CJ, Paul K, et al: Minimally invasive diagnosis of renal artery stenosis by spiral computed tomography angiography. Kidney Int 1995;48:1332–1337.

7. Elkohen M, Beregi JP, et al: A prospective study of helical computed tomography angiography versus angiography for the detection of renal artery stenoses in hypertensive patients. J Hypertens 1996;14:525–528.

8. Borello JA, Li D, et al: Renal arteries: Clinical comparison of three-dimensional time-of-flight MR angiographic sequences and radiographic angiography. Radiology 1995; 197:793–799.

9. de Haan MW, Kouwenhoven M, et al: Renovascular disease in patients with hypertension: Detection with systolic and diastolic gating in three-dimensional, phase-contrast MR angiography. Radiology 1996;198:449–456.

10. Gilfeather M, Yoon H, Siegelman ES, et al: Renal artery stenosis: Evalution with conventional angiography versus gadolinium-enhanced MR angiography. Radiology 1999; 210:367–372.

11. Black HR, Nally JV (eds): The role of captopril scintigraphy in the diagnosis and management of renovascular hypertension: A consensus conference. Am J Hypertens 1991; 4(Suppl):661S–751S.

12. Setaro JF, Chen CC, Hoffer PB, Black HR: Captopril renography in the diagnosis of renal artery stenosis and the prediction of improvement with revascularization: The Yale vascular center experience. Am J Hypertens 1991;4(Suppl):698S–705S.

13. Black HR: Captopril renal scintigraphy—a way to distinguish functional from anatomic renal artery stenosis. J Nucl Med 1992;33:2045–2046.

Medications Commonly Used in the Treatment of Hypertension

APPENDIX V

Medications Commonly Used in the Treatment of Hypertension

Medication			Dosage			Side Effects		Availability		
Class/Drug	Brand Names	Start Dose	Adjustment Intervals	Maximum Dosages	Frequent	Infrequent		Dose Sizes	Tablet or Capsule	Scored
Thiazide diuretics										
Hydrochloro- thiazide	HydroDiuril and others	12.5 mg once daily	2–3 weeks	25 mg/day	Impotence Hypokalemia Hypomagnesemia Hyperuricemia Hyperglycemia Hyperlipidemia (transient) Mild metabolic alkalosis Hyponatremia Ineffective in renal failure (except metolazone)	Acute interstitial nephritis Blood dyscrasias Rash		25, 50, 100 mg	Tab	Yes
Indapamide	Lozol	1.25–2.5 mg once daily	2 weeks	2.5 mg/day	Same as thiazides without hyperlipidemia	Same as other thiazides		1.25, 2.5 mg	Tab	No
Metolazone	Diulo Zaroxolyn	1.25 mg once daily	2 weeks	10 mg/day	Same as other thiazides but effective in renal failure	Same as other thiazides		2.5, 5, 10 mg	Tab	No
Loop diuretics (Effective in renal failure)										
Furosemide	Lasix	20 mg twice daily	2 weeks	600 mg/day	Impotence Hypokalemia Hypomagnesemia Hyperuricemia Hyperglycemia Hyperlipidemia Metabolic alkalosis Hypernatremia	Hyponatremia Hypocalcemia Blood dyscrasia Rash Acute interstitial nephritis Thromboembolism		20, 40, 80 mg	Tab	Yes (except 20 mg)
Ethacrynic acid	Edecrin	12.5 mg twice daily	3 weeks	400 mg/day	Same as furosemide	Same as furosemide		25, 50 mg	Tab	Yes

Bumetanide	Bumex	0.25 mg twice daily	3 weeks	10 mg/day	Same as furosemide	Same as furosemide	0.5, 1, 2 mg	Tab	No
Torsemide	Demadex	2.5 mg once daily	3 weeks(?)	200 mg/day	Same as furosemide	Same as furosemide	5, 10, 20, 100 mg	Tab	Yes
Potassium-sparing diuretics (Main use to prevent or correct hypokalemia)									
Spironolactone	Aldactone	25 mg once daily	—	400 mg/day	Hyperkalemia Gastrointestinal disturbances Gynecomastia	Rash Hyponatremia Agranulocytosis	25, 50, 100 mg	Tab	Only 100s
Triamterene	Dyrenium	50 mg once daily	—	200 mg/day	Hyperkalemia Gastrointestinal disturbances Not antihypertensive	Triamterene kidney stones	50, 100 mg	Tab	No
Amiloride	Midamor	5 mg once daily	—	10 mg/day	Hyperkalemia Gastrointestinal disturbances Headache	Rash	5 mg	Tab	No
Central alpha-2 agonists									
Clonidine	Catapres	0.1 mg twice daily	3 days	2.4 mg/day	Dry mouth Urinary retention Somnolence	Sodium retention Insomnia	0.1, 0.2, 0.3 mg	Tab	No
	Catapres TTS patches	2.5 mg every week (TTS-1)	14 days	2 TTS-3 patches (15 mg) weekly	Worsening AV block Bradycardia Fatigue Rash with patches		TTS: 2.5, 5, 7.5 mg	Patch	—
Methyldopa	Aldomet	250 mg twice daily	3 days	2000 mg/day	Somnolence Worsening AV block Bradycardia Fatigue Orthostasis Positive Coombs test	Hepatitis* Hemolysis	125, 250, 500 mg	Tab	No
Guanabenz	Wytensin	4 mg twice daily	—	16 mg twice daily	Same as clonidine	Same as clonidine	4, 8, 16 mg	Tab	No
Guanfacine	Tenex	1 mg once daily	2 weeks	3 mg once daily	Same as clonidine	Same as clonidine	1, 2 mg	Tab	No

* Stop methyldopa for abnormal liver function or hemolytic anemia but not just for positive Coombs test.

Continued on following page

Medications Commonly Used in the Treatment of Hypertension (*Continued*)

Medication			Dosage			Side Effects		Availability		
Class/Drug	Brand Names	Start Dose	Adjustment Intervals	Maximum Dosage	Frequent	Infrequent		Dose Sizes	Tablet or Capsule	Scored
Nonselective alpha blockers										
Phenoxybenzamine	Dibenzyline	10 mg twice daily	2 days	Over 120 mg	Postural hypotension Tachycardia Impotence Nasal congestion	GI upset Fatigue Drowsiness		10 mg	Cap	No
Peripheral alpha-1 blockers (arteriolar and venous dilators)										
Prazosin	Minipress	1 mg nightly then twice daily	2 weeks	20 mg/day	First-dose orthostasis Dizziness Fatigue Headache Somnolence	Leukopenia		1, 2, 5 mg	Cap	No
Terazosin	Hytrin	Same as prazosin, but once daily	2 weeks	20 mg/day	Same as prazosin	Same as prazosin		1, 2, 5, 10 mg	Cap	No
Doxazosin	Cardura	Same as prazosin, but once daily	2 weeks	16 mg/day	Same as prazosin	Same as prazosin		1, 2, 4, 8 mg	Tab	No
Nonselective beta blockers without ISA[†]										
Propranolol	Inderal	20 mg two or three times daily	2–4 weeks	1000 mg/day	Fatigue Exacerbation of asthma Masking of hyperglycemia Delay of recovery from hypoglycemia Worsening of hypertension during hypoglycemia Impotence Worsening of Raynaud's Worsening of arterial insufficiency (?) Reduction of renal blood flow Negative inotropic and chronotropic effects Worsening of hyperlipidemia			10, 20, 30, 40, 80 mg	Tab	Yes
	Inderal-LA	LA 80 mg once or twice daily						LA: 80, 120 160 mg		

Nadolol	Corgard	40 mg once daily	2–4 weeks	480 mg/day	Same as propranolol	20, 40, 80, 120, 160 mg	Tab	Yes
Timolol	Blocadren	10 mg twice daily	2–4 weeks	60 mg/day	Same as propranolol	5, 10, 20 mg	Tab	Yes (except 5 mg)

Nonselective beta blockers with ISA†
(Preferred for patients with symptomatic bradycardia; do not affect serum lipids; may not reduce mortality after myocardial infarction like non-ISA drugs.)

Pindolol	Visken	5 mg twice daily	2–4 weeks	60 mg/day	Like propranolol, except • Less chronotropic effect • No reduction in renal blood flow • No adverse effects on blood lipid levels	5, 10 mg	Tab	No
Penbutolol	Levatol	10 mg once daily	2–4 weeks	20 mg/day	Same as pindolol	20 mg	Long tab	No

Beta-1 selective blockers without ISA†
(Selective only in low doses; may be preferred for diabetics since they may not delay recovery from hypoglycemia and are less likely to exacerbate hypertension during hypoglycemia.)

Atenolol	Tenormin	50 mg once daily	2–4 weeks	100 mg/day	In low dose: • Fatigue • Depression • Impotence • Negative chronotropic and inotropic effects In higher doses: • All of nonselective effects (like propranolol, including lowering high-density lipoproteins)	25, 50, 100 mg	Tab	Only 50 mg

Continued on following page

† ISA = intrinsic sympathomimetic activity.

Medications Commonly Used in the Treatment of Hypertension (*Continued*)

| Medication | | Dosage | | | Side Effects | | | Availability | |
Class/Drug	Brand Names	Start Dose	Adjustment Intervals	Maximum Dosage	Frequent	Infrequent	Dose Sizes	Tablet or Capsule	Scored
Beta-1 selective blockers without ISA† (*Cont.*)									
Metoprolol	Lopressor	50 mg twice daily	2–4 weeks	400 mg/day	Like atenolol *plus* elevates blood levels of verapamil		50, 100 mg	Long tab	No
	Toprol-XL	25–50 mg once daily					50, 100 200 mg	Tab	Yes
Betaxolol	Kerlone	5–10 mg once daily	2–4 weeks	20 mg/day	Like metoprolol *plus* headache, but no adverse effect on high-density lipoproteins		10, 20 mg	Tab	Only 10 mg
Bisoprolol	Zebeta	2.5–5 mg once daily	2 weeks	20 mg/day	Like atenolol *plus* diarrhea		5, 10 mg	Tab	Only 5 mg
Beta-1 selective blocker with ISA†									
Acebutolol	Sectral	200 mg once daily	2–4 weeks	600 mg/day	Fatigue Depression Impotence Loses beta-1 selectivity at higher doses		200, 400 mg	Cap	No
Combined alpha-1 and beta blocker with ISA†									
Labetalol	Trandate Normodyne	200 mg twice daily	3 days	2400 mg/day(?)	Bronchospasm Fatigue Severe orthostasis Impotence Paresthesias Nonselective at higher doses	Hepatitis Lupus Tremor	100, 200, 300 mg	Cap	No
Combined alpha-1 and beta blocker without ISA†									
Carvedilol	Coreg	6.25 mg twice daily	2 weeks	50 mg	Bronchospasm Fatigue				

Carvedilol *(Cont.)*

Severe orthostasis
Impotence
Paresthesias
Worsening congestive heart failure

Nondihydropyridine calcium channel blockers

Generic	Brand	Dose	Titration	Max	Adverse effects	Additional effects	Strengths	Form	ISA[†]
Diltiazem	Cardizem	30 mg three times daily	4 weeks	540 mg/day	Moderately negative inotropic effects		30, 60, 90, 120 mg	Tab	Yes (except 30 mg)
	Cardizem SR	60 mg twice daily			Mild SA and AV conduction disturbances		60, 90, 120 mg	Cap	
	Cardizem CD	180 mg once daily			Increased digoxin levels		180, 240, 300 mg	Cap	
	Dilacor XR	180 mg once daily			Constipation		120, 180, 240 mg	Cap	
	Tiazac	120 mg once daily			Mild edema		120, 180, 240 300, 360, 420 mg	Cap	
					Use beta blocker with caution				
Verapamil	Calan	40 mg three times daily	4 weeks	480 mg/day	Most negatively inotropic effects	Gingival hyperplasia	40, 80, 120 mg	Cap	Yes (except 40 mg)
	Calan SR	120 mg once or twice daily			Greatest AV block		120, 180, 240 mg	Tab	Yes (except 120 mg)
	Verelan	120 mg once or twice daily			Most constipating		120, 180, 240 mg	Cap	No
	Isoptin						40, 80, 120 mg	Tab	Yes
	Isoptin SR						120, 180, 240 mg	Tab	Yes (except 120 mg)
	Covera-HS	180 QHS	1–2 weeks				180, 240 mg	N/A	N/A
	Verelan PM	100–200 mg QHS					100, 200, 300 mg	N/A	N/A

Dihydropyridine calcium channel blockers

Generic	Brand	Dose	Titration	Max	Adverse effects	Additional effects	Strengths	Form	ISA[†]
Nifedipine	Procardia XL	30 mg once daily	4 weeks	120 mg/day	Tachycardia	Gingival hyperplasia	30, 60, 90 mg	Cap	No
	Adalat CC				Headache			Tab	No
					Local edema				
					Orthostasis				
					Mildly negative inotropic effects				
					Flushing				

Continued on following page

[†] ISA = intrinsic sympathomimetic activity.

Medications Commonly Used in the Treatment of Hypertension (*Continued*)

Medication			Dosage			Side Effects		Availability		Scored
Class/Drug	Brand Names	Start Dose	Adjustment Intervals	Maximum Dosage	Frequent	Infrequent		Dose Sizes	Tablet or Capsule	
Dihydropyridine calcium channel blockers (*Cont.*)										
Nicardipine	Cardene	20 mg three times daily	4 weeks	120 mg/day	Tachycardia Local edema Headache	Gingival hyperplasia		20, 30 mg	Cap	No
	Cardene SR	30 mg twice daily						30, 45, 60 mg	Cap	No
Felodipine	Plendil	5 mg once daily	3 weeks	10 mg/day	Same as nicardipine			5, 10 mg	Tab	No
Amlodipine	Norvasc	2.5 mg once daily	2–66 weeks	10 mg/day	Same as nicardapine			2.5, 5, 10 mg	Tab	No
Isradipine	DynaCirc	2.5 mg twice daily	4 weeks	10 mg/day	Same as nicardipine			2.5, 5 mg	Cap	No
Nisoldipine	Sular	10–20 mg once daily	1–2 weeks	60 mg/day	Same as nicardipine			10, 20, 30, 40 mg	Tab	No
Nitrendipine		10 mg once daily, twice daily dosing thereafter		40 mg/day	Same as nicardipine					
Direct-acting vasodilators										
Hydralazine	Apresoline	10–20 mg two to four times daily	1 week	300–400 mg/day	Tachycardia[‡] Fluid retention Angina Headache Positive antinuclear antibodies	Lupus Nasal congestion Rash Hepatitis Glomerulonephritis		10, 25, 50, 100 mg	Tab	No
Minoxidil	Loniten	5 mg once daily	4 days	80 mg/day	Tachycardia[‡] Fluid retention Angina Hypertrichosis Coarse facial features (like acromegaly)	Pericardial effusion Hypopericardium Pulmonary fibrosis Cytopenias		2.5, 10 mg	Tab	Yes

Angiotensin-converting enzyme inhibitors

Generic	Brand	Dose	Time	Max dose	Adverse effects	Adverse effects	Strengths	Form	Scored
Captopril	Capoten	12.5 mg twice daily or three daily	2 weeks	150 mg/day	Cough Flushing Hyperkalemia Dysgeusia Orthostasis Azotemia in patients with congestive heart failure or renal artery stenosis or some patients with pre-existing nephrosclerosis	Azotemia Angioedema Cytopenias Erythroderma Membranous nephropathy	12.5, 25, 37.5, 50, 100 mg	Tab	Only 12.5 mg
Enalapril	Vasotec	2.5 mg twice daily	1–2 weeks	60–80 mg/day	Same as captopril	Same as captopril	2.5, 5, 10, 20 mg	Tab	Only 2.5 and 5 mg
Lisinopril	Zestril Prinivil	10 mg once to twice daily or 5 mg twice daily	2–4 weeks	60–80 mg/day	Same as captopril	Same as captopril	5, 10, 20, 40 mg	Tab	Only 5 mg
Ramipril	Altace	1.25–2.5 mg once to twice daily	2–4 weeks	40 mg/day	Same as captopril	Same as captopril	1.25, 2.5, 5, 10 mg	Cap	No
Benazepril	Lotensin	5–10 mg once to twice daily	2–4 weeks	40–80 mg/day	Same as captopril	Same as captopril	5, 10, 20, 40 mg	Tab	No
Fosinopril	Monopril	10 mg once to twice daily	2–4 weeks	80 mg/day	Same as captopril	Same as captopril	10, 20 mg	Tab	No
Quinapril	Accupril	10 mg once to twice daily	2–4 weeks	80 mg/day	Same as captopril	Same as captopril	5, 10, 20, 40 mg	Tab	Yes
Moexipril	Univasc	3.75–7.5 mg once to twice daily AC	2–4 weeks	60 mg/day (15 for CCR < 40)	Same as captopril	Same as captopril	7.5, 15 mg	Tab	Yes
Trandolapril	Mavik	0.5–2 mg once daily	1–2 weeks	8 mg/day	Same as captopril	Same as captopril	1, 2, 4 mg	Tab	Only 1 mg

Continued on following page

‡The common adverse effects of tachycardia, angina, and fluid retention seen with either hydralazine or minoxidil are usually largely preventable through the concurrent use of diuretics and either beta blockers or central agents.

Medications Commonly Used in the Treatment of Hypertension (*Continued*)

| Medication | | Dosage | | | Side Effects | | Availability | | |
Class/Drug	Brand Names	Start Dose	Adjustment Intervals	Maximum Dosage	Frequent	Infrequent	Dose Sizes	Tablet or Capsule	Scored
Angiotensin II receptor antagonists									
Losartan	Cozaar	25–50 mg	3–6 weeks	100 mg/day	Muscle cramps Backache Postural hypotension Nasal congestion Sinusitis Probably azotemia in patients with congestive heart failure or renal artery stenosis or some patients with preexisting nephro-sclerosis	Hyperkalemia Angioedema Serious dermatologic reactions Abnormal liver function tests	25, 50 mg	Tab	No
Valsartan	Diovan	80 mg once daily	4 weeks	320 mg/day	Same as losartan	Same as losartan	80, 160 mg	Cap	No
Irbesartan	Avapro	75–150 mg once daily	4 weeks	300 mg/day	Same as losartan	Same as losartan	75, 150, 300	Tab	No
Candesartan	Atacand	2–16 mg once daily	4–6 weeks	32 mg/day	Same as losartan	Same as losartan	4, 8, 16, 32 mg	Tab	No
Telmisartan	Micardis	40 mg once daily	4–6 weeks	80 mg/day	Same as losartan	Same as losartan	40, 80 mg	Tab	Yes
Postganglionic blockers									
Guanethidine	Ismelin	10 mg once daily	1–2 weeks	300 mg/day	Diarrhea Postural hypotension Syncope Fluid retention Nausea Vomiting	Parotid gland tenderness Congestive heart failure Ptosis Myalgia	10, 25 mg	Tab	Yes

Guanethidine (*Cont.*)

					Side effects		Strength	Form	ISA
					Dry mouth Blurred vision Fatigue Depression Impaired ejaculation Precipitation of asthma Edema Angina Urinary incontinence Nocturia Nasal stuffiness	Dermatitis Alopecia Blood dyscrasia Priapism Azotemia			
Guanadrel	Hylorel	5 mg twice daily	1 week	150 mg/day	Same as guanethidine ? Less severe	Same as guanethidine	10, 25 mg	Tab	Yes
Reserpine	Serpasil	0.05 mg once daily	3 weeks	1 mg/day	Depression Drowsiness Nasal congestion Weight gain Abdominal cramps Diarrhea Fluid retention Dyspepsia Exacerbation of peptic ulcer Impotence Bronchospasm	Extrapyramidal effects	0.1, 0.25 mg	Tab	No

* Stop methyldopa for abnormal liver function or hemolytic anemia but not just for positive Coombs test.

† ISA = intrinsic sympathomimetic activity.

‡ The common adverse effects of tachycardia, angina, and fluid retention seen with either hydralazine or minoxidil are usually largely preventable through the concurrent use of diuretics and either beta blockers or central agents.

APPENDIX V
(Supplement)

Common Combination Antihypertensive Drugs*

Medication			Availability	
Class/Drug	Brand Names	Dose Sizes	Tablet or Capsule	Scored
Combination diuretics				
Hydrochlorothiazide/spironolactone*	Aldactazide	25/25 mg	Tab	No
		50/50 mg	Tab	Yes
Hydrochlorothiazide/triamterene*	Dyazide	25/37.5 mg	Cap	No
	Maxzide-25	25/37.5 mg	Tab	Yes
	Maxzide	50/75 mg	Tab	Yes
Hydrochlorothiazide/amiloride*	Moduretic	50/5 mg	Tab	Yes
Diuretic/nonselective beta blockers				
Hydrochlorothiazide/propranolol*	Inderide	25/40 and 25/80 mg	Tab	Yes
	Inderide-LA	50/80, 50/120 and 50/160 mg	Caps	No
Hydrochlorothiazide/timolol	Timolide	25/10 mg	Tab	No
Diuretic/selective beta-1 blockers				
Chlorthalidone/atenolol	Tenoretic	25/50 and 25/100 mg	Tab	Yes (only 25/50)
Hydrochlorthiazide/bisoprolol	Ziac	6.25/2.5, 6.25/5, 6.25/10 mg	Tab	No
Hydrochlorthiazide/metoprolol	Lopressor HCT	25/50, 25/100, 50/100 mg	Long tab	Yes
Diuretic/alpha-2 blockers				
Polythiazide/prazosin	Minizide	0.5/1, 0.5/2, 0.5/5 mg	Cap	No
Diuretic/ACE inhibitors				
Hydrochlorothiazide/captopril	Capozide	25/15, 25/25, 50/15 and 50/50 mg	Tab	No
Hydrochlorothiazide/enalapril	Vaseretic	25/10 mg	Tab	No
Hydrochlorothiazide/lisinopril	Zestoretic Prinzide	12.5/20 and 25/20 mg	Tab	No
Hydrochlorothiazide/benazepril	Lotensin HCT	6.25/5, 12.5/10, 12.5/20, and 25/20 mg	Tab	Yes
Hydrochlorothiazide/moexipril	Uniretic	12.5/7.5 and 25/15 mg	Tab	Yes
Diuretic/central agents				
Hydrochlorothiazide/methyldopa*	Aldoril	15/250, 25/250, 30/500 and 50/500 mg	Tab	No
Chlorothiazide/methyldopa	Aldoclor	150/250 and 250/250 mg	Tab	No

Continued on facing page

Common Combination Antihypertensive Drugs (*Continued*)*

Medication		Availability		
Class/Drug	Brand Names	Dose Sizes	Tablet or Capsule	Scored
Diuretic/central agents (*Cont.*)				
Chlorthalidone/clonidine*	Combipres	15/0.1, 15/0.2, and 15/0.3 mg	Tab	Yes
Diuretic/vasodilators				
Hydrochlorothiazide/hydralazine	Apresazide	25/25, 50/50, and 50/100 mg	Cap	No
Diuretic/postganglionic inhibitors				
Chlorthalidone/reserpine	Regroton	50/0.25 mg	Tab	No
	Demi-Regroton	25/0.25 mg		
Chlorothiazide/reserpine*	Diupres	250/0.125 mg 500/0.125 mg	Tab	Yes
Hydrochlorothiazide reserpine*	Hydropres	25/0.125 mg	Tab	Yes
Hydroflumethiazide/reserpine*	Salutensin-Demi	25/0.125 mg	Tab	No
	Salutensin	50/0.125 mg	Tab	Yes
Hydrochlorothiazide/guanethidine	Esimil	2.5/100 mg	Tab	Yes
Diuretic/vasodilator/postganglionic inhibitor				
Hydrochlorothiazide/hydralazine/ reserpine	Ser-Ap-Es	15/25/0.1 mg	Tab	No
Diuretic/angiotensin II blockers				
Hydrochlorothiazide/losartan	Hyzaar	12.5/50 mg	Tab	No
		25/100 mg	Tab	No
Hydrochlorothiazide/valsartan	Diovan HCT	12.5/80 mg 12.5/160 mg	Tab	No
Hydrochlorothiazide/irbesartan	Avalide	12.5/150 mg 12.5/300 mg	Tab	No
Calcium channel blocker/ACE inhibitors				
Amlodipine/benazepril	Lotrel	2.5/10, 5/10, and 5/20 mg	Cap	No
Verapamil/trandolapril	Tarka	180/2, 240/1, 240/2 and 240/4 mg	Tab	No
Diltiazem/enalapril	Teczem	180/5 mg (max of 3 tabs/day)	Tab	No
Felodipine/enalapril	Lexxel	5/5 mg (max of 2 tabs/day)	Tab	No

Generally, combination drugs are reserved for use in patients who have been titrated to similar or identical doses of individual drugs first. In such patients they may be less costly and more convenient and therefore increase compliance. Hydrochlorothiazide/bisoprolol is the only fixed-dose drug combination approved by the FDA for initial therapy as of the time of this writing.
* Denotes drugs available as generic.

Dosage Adjustments in Renal Impairment

APPENDIX VI

Dosage Adjustments in Renal Impairment[1,2]

I. **Medications that Usually Do Not Require Adjustment with Renal Insufficiency**
   A. **Diuretics**
      1. Furosemide
      2. Metolazone
      3. Bumetanide
   B. **Central agents**
      1. Clonidine
      2. Guanabenz
      3. Guanfacine
   C. **Alpha blockers**
      1. Prazosin
      2. Doxazosin
      3. Terazosin
   D. **Beta blockers***
      1. Nonselective without ISA
         a. Propranolol
         b. Timolol
      2. Beta-1 selective without ISA—metoprolol
      3. Nonselective with ISA
         a. Penbutol
         b. Pindolol
      4. Combined beta-1 and alpha blocker: labetalol
   E. **Angiotensin-converting enzyme (ACE) inhibitors***
      1. Fosinopril
      2. Trandolapril
      3. Ramipril
   F. **Angiotensin receptor blockers**—all
   G. **Direct vasodilator**—minoxidil
   H. **Calcium channel blockers**—all
   I. **Nitrates**—all
II. **Antihypertensive Agents Generally Contraindicated or Ineffective in Renal Failure**
   A. All potassium-conserving diuretics
   B. Acetazolamide
   C. Indapamide
   D. Thiazides (except metolazone)
   E. High-dose ACE inhibitors
III. **Drugs to be Used Only with Caution in Patients with Renal Impairment**
   A. Beta blockers, ACE inhibitors, and angiotensin receptor blockers
      1. Monitor renal function and potassium closely
      2. Discontinue, if possible, in patients with significant hyperkalemia
      3. ACE inhibitors are contraindicated in anyone with history of hyperkalemia

---

* Use beta blockers and/or ACE inhibitors in renal failure with extreme caution, especially in combination, because of danger of hyperkalemia.

B. Nitroprusside
   1. Although dosage is unchanged, toxic metabolites accumulate sooner
   2. Monitor levels of thiocyanate closely if used for more than 24–48 hours
C. Nonselective beta blockers with ISA
   1. Significant risk of prolonged hypoglycemia in diabetics
   2. Significant risk of spontaneous or worsened hyperkalemia
   3. May reduce renal blood flow
D. Methyldopa
   1. Long-acting metabolites persist for days
   2. Orthostatic hypotension limits usefulness, especially in uremia

REFERENCES

1. Physicians' Desk Reference, 53rd ed. New Jersey, Medical Economics Co., 1999.
2. Bakris GL: Drug dosages for patients with renal failure. In Stein JH (ed): Internal Medicine: Diagnosis and Therapy, 3rd ed. Norwalk, CN, Appleton & Croft, 1993, pp 352–387.
3. Bennet WM, Aronoff GR, Golper TA, et al: Drug Prescribing in Renal Failure, 2nd ed. Philadelphia, American College of Physicians, 1991.
4. Schrier RW, Gambertoglio JG (eds): Handbook of Drug Therapy in Liver and Kidney Disease. Boston, Little, Brown, 1991.

Side Effects of Antihypertensive Medications

APPENDIX VII

Side Effects of Antihypertensive Medications

TABLE A16.   Relatively Benign and Non–Life-Threatening Drug Reactions

Symptom/Condition	Possibly Beneficial Drugs	Possibly Harmful Drugs
Headache	Calcium channel blockers Central agents Beta blockers	Hydralazine Alpha blockers Calcium channel blockers
Hot flashes	Clonidine	Calcium channel blockers
Anxiety	Beta blockers Central agents Reserpine	
Lethargy		Central agents Beta blockers
Impotence	ACE inhibitors	All except ACE inhibitors
Constipation	Guanethidine	Calcium channel blockers Diuretics Central agents Trimethaphan
Diarrhea	Calcium channel blockers Diuretics Central agents	Reserpine Guanethidine
Essential tremor	Beta blockers	Alpha blockers
Baldness	Minoxidil	Hydralazine
Rhinorrhea or tearing	Clonidine	Beta blockers
Raynaud's phenomenon	Nifedipine Felodipine Diltiazem Reserpine Alpha-1 blockers ACE inhibitors[4] (?)	Beta blockers
Edema	Diuretics Beta blockers (?) ACE inhibitors	Alpha blockers Calcium channel blockers Hydralazine Minoxidil Methyldopa
Insomnia	Central agents	

TABLE A17.   Potentially Serious Adverse Drug Reactions

Condition/ Symptom	Drugs Possibly Beneficial	Drugs Possibly Harmful	Contraindicated
Isolated systolic hypertension	Diuretics Beta blockers Long-acting CCBs Long-acting nitrates Alpha blockers		
Asthma	Dihydropyridine CCBs	High-dose diuretics ACE inhibitors All alpha agents	Beta blockers (all)
Diabetes*	ACE inhibitors* Heart rate-lowering CCBs	High-dose diuretics High-dose CCBs	Beta blockers (nonselective)

Continued on facing page

TABLE A17. Potentially Serious Adverse Drug Reactions *(Continued)*

Condition/ Symptom	Drugs Possibly Beneficial	Drugs Possibly Harmful	Contraindicated
Tachyarrhythmias	Beta blockers Heart rate-lowering CCBs Central agents	Hydralazine[†] Nifedipine[†]	
Bradyarrhythmias	Hydralazine	Central agents Beta blockers Mifebradil	
Heart block		Diltiazem	Verapamil Beta blockers Mibefradil
Renal insufficiency	ACE inhibitors* CCBs Alpha blockers Metolazone Loop diuretics	ACE inhibitors Diazoxide Nonselective beta blockers Nitroprusside	Thiazides (except metolazone)
Bilateral or solitary renal artery stenosis	CCBs Beta blockers	ACE inhibitors	
Left ventricular hypertrophy	CCBs Beta blockers Central agents Diuretics[§] ACE inhibitors		
Hyperlipidemia	Alpha blockers CCBs	Beta blocker without ISA[‡] Diuretics	
Hyperkalemia	Diuretics (not potassium retaining) CCBs[//]	Potassium-retaining diuretics Beta blockers[§] ACE inhibitors	
Depression		Beta blockers Reserpine Central alpha agonists (antagonized by tricyclics) ACE inhibitors if taking lithium	Diuretics if taking lithium
Angina	Beta blockers CCBs	Diuretics	Hydralazine (without beta blockade) Guanethidine Minoxidil (without beta blockade)
Congestive heart failure	Diuretics ACE inhibitors Amlodipine (?) Angiotensin receptor antagonists	Beta blockers Diltiazem Other CCBs	Verapamil
After myocardial infarction	Beta blockers (without ISA) Heart rate-lowering CCBs ACE inhibitors	Hydralazine	

Continued on following page

TABLE A17. Potentially Serious Adverse Drug Reactions *(Continued)*

Condition/ Symptom	Drugs Possibly Beneficial	Drugs Possibly Harmful	Contraindicated
Orthostasis or cerebral ischemia	Beta blockers Clonidine	Labetalol Guanethidine Diuretics Methyldopa ACE inhibitors (especially with diuretics)	
Pregnancy	Methyldopa	Some beta blockers (?) Diuretics	ACE inhibitors Ganglionic blockers Nitroprusside (avoid if possible)
Pheochromocytoma	Peripheral alpha blockers Heart rate-lowering CCBs		Minoxidil Beta blockers (without alpha blockade)
AV block or bradycardia	Hydralazine	Guanethidine Central agents Reserpine	Beta blockers Verapamil Diltiazem
Liver disease	Nonselective beta blockers for varices	Methyldopa Labetalol Hydralazine	
Systemic lupus erythematosus			Hydralazine Methyldopa Acebutolol

CCBs = calcium channel blockers.

* ACE inhibitors and CCBs or both together slow the progression of **early** diabetic renal disease, but both (particularly ACE inhibitors) may worsen renal disease under certain circumstances (see Chapter 4). There is a significant risk of serious hyperkalemia in patients with renal impairment, especially diabetics in whom ACE inhibitors are used. Twenty-four hour urine protein determinations **must** be obtained before and during the use of ACE inhibitors in such patients. Serum creatinine also should be checked during the first week of therapy and frequently thereafter.

† Reflex tachycardia is common.

‡ Beta blockers with ISA and at least one beta-1 selective beta blocker (betaxolol) do not seem to affect lipid profiles adversely.

§ Worsening or new-onset hyperlipidemia may not occur with certain diuretics and often is transient when it does occur. In some cases, alpha blockers have been reported to reverse elevations in lipids accompanying drug usage.

‖ Directly inhibit aldosterone release.

REFERENCES

1. Pierce DM: A review of the clinical pharmacokinetics and metabolism of the alpha 1-adrenergic antagonist indoramin. Xenobiotica 1990;20:1357–1367.
2. Challenor VF: Angiotensin converting enzyme inhibitors in Raynaud's phenomenon. Drugs 1994;48:864–867.
3. Neaton JD, Grimm RH, Prineas RJ, et al: Treatment of mild hypertension study: Final results. JAMA 1993;270:713–724.
4. Frohlich ED, Horinaka S: Cardiac and aortic effects of angiotensin converting enzyme inhibitors. Hypertension 1991;18(Suppl II):II-2–II-7.

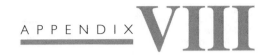

APPENDIX VIII

Important Drug Interactions

APPENDIX VIII

Important Drug Interactions[1–3]*

Drug	Second Drug	Reaction	Comments
Beta blockers or labetalol	Central alpha agents (e.g., methyldopa,) clonidine)	Severe paradoxical hypertension	Taper other to zero 3 days before new drug; avoid concurrent use; should not be used in combination; no additional pressure lowering
	Peripheral alpha blockers	Exaggerated first-dose hypotension Orthostasis	Lower initial dose
	Calcium channel blockers	Conduction defects	Less with dihydropyridines (e.g., nifedipine)
	Hydralazine	Increased beta blockade	
	Thiazides	Greater hyperglycemia	More severe with hypokalemia
	NSAIDs	Impaired antihypertensive effect	Avoid this class
		Hyperkalemia	Especially with renal insufficiency or other interacting drugs
		Worsening renal function	Avoid this combination in renal impairment
	ACE inhibitors	Hyperkalemia	Monitor potassium levels closely, especially in diabetics or renal impairment
	OTC adrenergic agonists	Hypertension	Due to unopposed alpha stimulation; avoid
Carvedilol	Digoxin	Increased digoxin levels	Monitor digoxin levels
	Cimetidine	Increased serum levels of carvedilol	Start with lower doses of carvedilol
	Rifampin	Markedly reduced serum levels of carvedilol	Avoid combination
	CYP2D6 inhibitors[†]	Increased levels of carvedilol	Start with lower doses of carvedilol
CCBs[4]	Peripheral alpha blockers	Hypotension	Use with care; avoid dihydropyridines
	Beta blockers	Congestive heart failure Conduction disturbances	Least for dihydropyridines, worst for verapamil
	Carbamazepine, rifampin, or phenobarbital	Decreased blood levels of CCBs Increased blood levels of anticonvulsants	Nifedipine may be less likely to interact, but other dihydropyridines (e.g., felodipine) do
	Cyclosporine	Increased cyclosporine levels	Watch levels closely if on verapamil or diltiazem
	Magnesium sulfate	Neuromuscular blockade Hypotension	Combination of these two drugs to treat preeclampsia is under study
	Fluoxetine	Exaggerated CCB effects	Use lower dose or avoid CCBs with flouxetine——especially verapamil
	Grapefruit juice	Exaggerated CCB effects	Use lower doses or avoid CCBs
	Cimetidine, ranitidine	Increased felodipine levels	Use lower doses

Continued on facing page

Important Drug Interactions* *(Continued)*

Drug	Second Drug	Reaction	Comments
CCBs *(cont.)*	Midazolam	Increased midazolam levels	Reduce midazolam dose
	Digoxin	Increased digoxin levels with verapamil	
	Quinidine	Increased quinidine levels with verapamil	
	Amiodarone	Worsening AV block with verapamil or diltiazem	
	Clonidine	Worsening AV block with verapamil or diltiazem	
	Rifampin, phenobarbital	Dramatically decreased CCB levels	
	Cyclosporine	Increased cyclosporine levels	Reduce cyclosporine dose; raise dose if mibefradil is stopped
ACE inhibitors	Lithium	High lithium levels	Use with extreme caution; monitor levels
	Diuretics	Hypotension	Taper off diuretics before using or use tiny doses initially
		Worsening renal function	Avoid this combination with bilateral renal artery stenosis or stenosis to solitary kidney
	Potassium-sparing diuretics	Hyperkalemia, especially with spironolactone	Avoid combination
	Beta blockers	Hyperkalemia	Monitor potassium levels, especially in diabetics
	NSAIDs	Hyperkalemia	Monitor potassium levels, especially in diabetics
		Renal insufficiency	Contraindicated combination, especially with renal impairment or hepatic dysfunction
	Antacids	Decreased bioavailability	Avoid concurrent administration
	Chlorpromazine, clozapine	Increased ACE inhibitor effect	
	Trimethoprim or trimethoprim sulfa	Hyperkalemia[5,6]	
	Heparin	Hyperkalemia[7]	
Methyldopa	Oral iron	Decreased methyldopa absorption[8]	
	Lithium	May increase lithium levels	
	Tricyclic antidepressants	May antagonize antihypertensive effect	
	Trifluoperazine	Severe hypertension	Prolongs half-life of catecholamines; avoid
	Beta blockers	Severe paradoxical hypertension, especially after methyldopa withdrawal	Taper other to zero by 3 days before starting new drug; avoid concurrent use; should not be used in combination; no additional pressure lowering

Continued on following page

Important Drug Interactions* *(Continued)*

Drug	Second Drug	Reaction	Comments
Clonidine	Monoamine oxidase inhibitors	Hallucinations	Avoid concurrent use if possible
	Haloperidol	Dementia	Stop both drugs if it occurs
	Diazoxide	Severe hypotension	Avoid concurrent use
	NSAIDs	Impaired antihypertensive effect	Avoid if possible
	Tricyclic antidepressants	May antagonize antihypertensive effect	Avoid
	Beta blockers	Severe paradoxical hypertension, especially after clonidine withdrawal	Taper other to zero by 3 days before starting new drug; avoid concurrent use; should not be used in combination; no additional pressure lowering
Alpha blockers	NSAIDs	Impaired antihypertensive effect	Avoid if possible
Diuretics	NSAIDs	Impaired antihypertensive effect; increased serum potassium with potassium-sparing diuretics	Avoid if possible
	Steroids	Impaired antihypertensive effect	Avoid if possible
	Lithium	Increased lithium levels	Avoid
	ACE inhibitors	Increased potassium with potassium-sparing diuretics	Use only with extreme caution
	Beta blockers	Increased potassium with potassium-sparing diuretics	Monitor potassium levels closely

Note: Impaired antihypertensive efficacy of all drugs except CCBs has been reported in patients taking most NSAIDs.

OTC = over-the-counter; CCBs = calcium channel blockers.

* Many potential hypertensive interactions are not listed here; one should consult a drug interaction handbook or (preferably) a computerized interaction database when scrutinizing medications in a hypertensive patient.

† Such as quinidine, fluoxetine, paroxetine, propafenone.

Additional Interactions Reported to Result in Severe Hypertension

1. Combination of amitriptyline, Sinemet, and metoclopramide[9]
2. Combination of doxepin, chlorpromazine, and guanethidine[10]
3. Levodopa (without carbidopa) and selegiline (or other monoamine oxidase inhibitors)[11–13]
4. Guanadrel, buspirone, and amantadine may cause hypertension in patients taking monoamine oxidase inhibitors

REFERENCES

1. Rizack MA, et al: The Medical Letter Drug Interaction Program for the IBM-PC. New Rochelle, NY, Medical Letter, 1993.
2. Rizack MA, Hillman CDM: The Medical Letter Handbook of Adverse Drug Interactions. New Rochelle, NY, Medical Letter, 1993.
3. Howes LG: Which drugs affect potassium? Drug Safety 1995;12:240–244.
4. Rosenthal T, Ezra D: Calcium antagonists drug interactions of clinical significance. Drug Safety 1995;13:157–187.

5. Bugge JF: Severe hyperkalemia induced by trimethoprim in combination with an angiotensin converting enzyme inhibitor in a patient with transplanted lungs. J Intern Med 1996;240:249–251.

6. Thomas RJ: Hyperkalemia and trimethoprim-sulfamethoxazole. Ann Intern Med 1996; 125:1015.

7. Durand D, Ader JL, et al: Inducing hyperkalemia by converting enzyme inhibitors and heparin. Kidney Int 1988;125(Suppl):S196–S197

8. Campbell N, Paddock V, Sundaram R: Alteration of methyldopa absorption, metabolism, and blood pressure control caused by ferrous sulfate and ferrous gluconate. Clin Pharmacol Ther 1988;43:381.

9. Rampton DS: Hypertensive crisis in a patient given Sinemet, metoclopramide, and amitriptyline. BMJ 1977;2:607–608.

10. Poe TE, Edwards JL, Taylor RB: Hypertensive crisis probably due to a drug interaction. Postgrad Med 1979;66:235–237.

11. Schildkraut JJ, et al: Biochemical and pressor effects of oral D,L-hydroxyphenylalanine in patients pretreated with antidepressant drugs. Ann NY Acad Sci 1963;107:1005.

12. Hunter KR: Monoamine oxidase inhibitors and L-dopa. BMJ 1970;3:388.

13. Baronti F, et al: Deprenyl effects on levodopa pharmacokinetics, mood, and free radical scavenging. Neurology 1992;42:541.

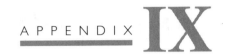

Parenteral Medications Used in the Treatment of Hypertension

APPENDIX IX

Parenteral Medications Used in the Treatment of Hypertension[1-4]

Class/Drug (Brand Name)	Medication		Dosage			Indications and Side Effects	
	Onset	Starting Dose*/Drip	Adjustment Interval and Usual Dose	Maximum Doses	Indications or Use	Side Effects[†]	
Diuretics							
Furosemide (Lasix)	15–60 min	20–80 mg intravenously	Usually 1–2 hr	600 mg/day or dose; give no faster than 20 mg/min when giving doses over 80 mg intravenously	Congestive heart failure (**not** for other hypertensive emergencies)	Deafness when given quickly	
Ethacrynic acid (Edecrin)	5 min	25 mg intravenously slowly	Variable, usually 1–2 hr	100 mg dose; slow push or by infusion	Congestive heart failure (**not** for other hypertensive emergencies)	Deafness when given quickly Phlebitis—avoid repeated injection in same peripheral site	
Beta blockers							
Propranolol (Inderal)	≤ 5 min	0.5 mg Do not exceed 1 mg/min injection rate	1 mg every 5 min until pulse pressure is < 60 mmHg or 0.15 mg/kg (10 mg) or significant bradycardia or heart block. Then 0.5–2 mg every 4–6 hr	Guided by response	Aortic dissection (with nitroprusside)	Bronchospasm, hypotension, bradycardia Requires constant ECG monitoring, especially during administration	
Metoprolol (Lopressor)	20 min	5 mg every 2 min to max of 15 mg	Repeat every 6 hr	60 mg	Pregnancy Aortic dissection (?)	Same as propranolol	
Esmolol (Brevibloc)	5 min	Load: 0.5 mg/kg over 1 min Drip: 0.05 mg/kg/min to start after	Repeat loading dose every 5 min as needed, while adjusting drip up, in 0.05 mg/kg/min increments	0.3 mg/kg/min	Beta-1 blockade **after** alpha blockade in operating room for excessive beta activity when removing a pheochromocytoma	Same as propranolol	

	Onset	Initial dose	Dosing/Titration	Maximum	Indications	Comments
Calcium channel blockers						
Nicardipine (Cardene I.V.)	Minutes	Drip: 0.1 mg-ml Start 50 ml/hr (5 mg/hr)	Increase by 25 ml/hr (2.5 mg/hr) every 15 min as needed Once controlled, reduce dose to 30 ml (3 mg/hr) Then titrate as needed	Maximum of 150 ml/hr (15 mg/hr)	Maintenance in N.P.O. patients May be used in heart failure and coronary artery disease May improve cardiac output in some patients with heart failure Usually improves coronary blood flow	Takes 45 min or more to reach steady state; Takes 30 min or more for effects to wane Lowers pressure more in hypertensive patients Tachycardia may occur Avoid with aortic stenosis or patients on cyclosporine May have negative inotropic effects, especially with beta blockers
Combined alpha and beta blockers						
Labetalol (Normodyne, Trandate)	5 min (bolus)	Bolus: 20 mg-intravenously Infusion: 800 mg/250 ml fluid (only after bolus)	Bolus: every 10 min to max of 300 mg Infusion (after initial bolus): 1–2 mg/min Adjust drip every 4–8 hr (long half-life) or discontinue for hypotension	300 mg boluses or 2400 mg/day infused	Early myocardial infarction Malignant hypertension Aortic dissection	Postural hypotension
Central alpha agonists						
Methyldopa (Aldomet)	4–6 hr	125–250 mg	125–500 mg every 4–12 hr	2000 mg/day	Intravenous maintenance or urgent therapy in patients unable to take oral medicine or be tube-fed	

Continued on following page

Parenteral Medications Used in the Treatment of Hypertension (*Continued*)[1-4]

Medication	Dosage		Indications and Side Effects			
Class/Drug (Brand Name)	Onset	Starting Dose*/Drip	Adjustment Interval and Usual Dose	Maximum Doses	Indications or Use	Side Effects[†]
Direct arteriolar vasodilators						
Hydralazine (Apresoline)	10 min intravenously	5 mg	5–20 mg intravenously (or up to 50 mg intramuscularly) if necessary) every 30 min	200 mg/day	Preeclampsia/ eclampsia	Headache Tachycardia Neonatal thrombocytopenia Angina
Diazoxide (Hyperstat)	5–15 min	30 mg Drip: 7.5–30 mg/min	30–150 mg every 5 min initially	5 mg/kg	Preeclampsia/ eclampsia	Fluid retention Tachycardia Hyperglycemia Dyspnea Cough Phlebitis (avoid nonintravenous administration) Angina Transient cerebrovascular ischemic attacks Stroke (with hypotension)
Arteriolar and venous vasodilators						
Nitroprusside (Nipride)	0.5–5 min	0.5 µg/kg/min (10 ml/hr) 50 mg in 250 ml of 5% dextrose in water	Every 5 min adjustments 1–3 µg/kg/min (20–40 ml/hr)	10 µg/kg/min (100 ml/hr of double strength or 50 ml/hr of quadruple strength)	Malignant hypertension With intravenous beta blocker for aortic dissection	Thiocyanate toxicity: tinnitus, blurred vision, delirium. Keep thiocyanate levels below 10; higher toxicity in renal insufficiency Cyanide toxicity: metabolic acidosis, resistance to hypotensive effect, dyspnea, vomiting, dizziness, ataxia. **Note:** thiocyanate levels do not correlate with cyanide levels; higher toxicity in hepatic insufficiency. Monitor anion gap and bicarbonate Discontinue for tachyphylaxis

Drug	Onset/Duration	Dose/Concentration	Titration interval	Toxic dose	Indication	Comments/Precautions	Side effects
Nitroglycerin (venous >> arteriolar)	≤ 5 min	3–6 µg/min (3–6 ml/hr) 25 mg in 250 ml of D5W = 100 mg/ml	5 min	≥ 200 µg/min	Hypertension with coronary ischemia	Avoid in inferior infarction if right ventricular function is impaired. Binds to polyvinyl chloride. Need special administration set	
Fenoldopam (Corlopam) (arterial)	Max at 15 minutes	0.1 µg/kg/min (No Bolus)	0.1 µg/kg/min every 15 min initially; less often as goal approached	1.6 µg/kg/min	Malignant hypertension, especially when renal and coronary blood flow maintenance are desirable. May be used with renal failure and at least moderate liver disease. May cause reflex tachycardia	Use beta blockers concurrently with extreme caution (excessive hypotension). May raise intraocular pressure and precipitate glaucoma. May cause hypokalemia. Contains sulfites. Has D1 agonist and alpha-2 antagonist activities. Limit use to 48 hr because of reflex tachycardia. Safety in coronary artery disease uncertain	
Ganglionic blockers							
Trimethaphan (Arfonad)		0.5–1 mg/min (15–30 ml/hr) 500 mg in 250 ml of 5% dextrose water or normal saline	0.5 mg/min (every 10 min)	≥ 6 mg/min (180 ml/hr or 90 ml/hr of double strength)	Aortic dissection		Tachycardia; Ileus; Dry mouth; Angina; Urinary retention; Pyrosis; Cycloplegia; Mydriasis; Urticaria (releases histamine); Tachyphylaxis

Continued on following page

Parenteral Medications Used in the Treatment of Hypertension (*Continued*)[1-4]

| Medication | Dosage | | Indications and Side Effects | | | |
Class/Drug (Brand Name)	Onset	Starting Dose*/Drip	Adjustment Interval and Usual Dose	Maximum Doses	Indications or Use	Side Effects[†]
Nonselective alpha blockers						
Phentolamine (Regitine)	≤ 5 min intravenously	5 mg intravenously or intramuscularly as needed			Pheochromocytoma Cocaine or amphetamine overdose unresponsive to sedation	Hypotension Myocardial infarction Stroke
ACE inhibitors						
Enalaprilat (Vasotec I.V.)	0.25–4 hr	0.625–1.25 mg over 5 min or more	1–6 hr 1.25 mg every 6 hr	20 mg/day	Parenteral maintenance Initiation of treatment	Excessive hypotension if patient is taking diuretics or is hypovolemic
Magnesium sulfate						
Magnesium sulfate	After loading	Load: 5 gm over 10 min Drip: 1 gm/hr	0.5–1.5 gm/hr Keep level 6–9 Judge doses clinically by reflexes		Toxemia	Paralysis Apnea (toxic doses)

* Doses in parentheses are average starting doses for a 70-kg patient.
† Also see Appendix X for further information about agents available orally.

REFERENCES

1. Black HR, Cohan JD, et al: The Sixth Report of the Joint National Committee on Detection, Evaluation, and Treatment of High Blood Pressure (JNC VI). Arch Intern Med 1997;157:2413–2445.
2. DeVault GA Jr: Therapy in hypertensive emergencies: A disease-specific approach. J Crit Ill 1991;6:477–484.
3. Calhoun DA, Oparil SO: Treatment of hypertensive crisis. N Engl J Med 1990;323: 1177–1184.
4. Gifford RW: Management of hypertensive crises. JAMA 1991;266:829–835.

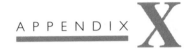

Nonparenteral Drugs Used for Treatment of Urgent Hypertension

APPENDIX X

Nonparenteral Drugs Used for Treatment of Urgent Hypertension*

Medication[†]	Initial Dose And Follow-up Dosing	Onset	Duration	Comments
Clonidine	0.2 mg, then 0.1 mg/hr to maximum of 0.6 mg total dose	30–60 min	6–12 hr	Good for clonidine withdrawal hypertension
Captopril	6.25–25 mg	15 min	2–6 hr	Risk of hypotension if patient is volume-depleted, taking diuretics, or has renal artery stenosis

* See Treatment of severe hypertension, p 70–72.

[†] Nifedipine (sublingual, oral, or crushed) is no longer considered appropriate for the treatment of urgent hypertension because of the risk of stroke and myocardial infarction

REFERENCE

Anderson RJ, Hart GR, Crumpler CP, et al: Oral clonidine loading in hypertensive urgencies. JAMA 1981;246:848–850.

Index